The tale of a BIG dog

A holistic guide to life with Hagrid

Rosie Lowry

TheTaleOfABigDog.com

Disclaimer

This is my story and how we live with our animals' best interests in mind. You will have your own set of circumstances with your animals. Together, my dogs and I chose the path we have been on and you're welcome to see what we did; it's unique to us. So this book tells a story of what we did. You may like a few of the ideas and might chose to find out more for yourself. You'll know your dog, your lifestyle and of course you'll have your own experiences and intuition about the appropriate steps to take. I would always say to anyone who lives and works with a dog to take time, invest in learning their language and how to read that in everyday circumstances. It takes time to practice, but being fluent in our dogs' communication is what animals deserve when they are part of our lives.

Lowry Industries
Ysgubor Celyn, Llanarmon Mynydd Mawr,
Llanrhaeadr ym Mochnant, Powys, Wales, SY10 0EB
www.laidbackdogs.com
Ordering Information: laidbackdogs@gmail.com.

ISBN: 978-0-9565934-2-9

Printed by Short Run Press in the United Kingdom. Graphic design: craftingwords.com

Contents

Acknowledgements

A HUGE THANK YOU to the adorable HAGRID who was a true gift and I am privileged that we shared our lives for a few years. He was the most wonderful, gentle, sensitive soul who continues to live on in my heart – so fondly remembered. I miss you so and while I didn't get everything right, that had always been my intention.

During the writing and moulding of this book I have been so fortunate to have met and worked with a whole team of amazingly lovely and talented people. Each one has added a magical something to this book, my life and I feel enriched in knowing each of you. It's been a fabulous journey; interesting, with all its twists and turns, and I thank you all for working alongside me although it's not always been straightforward, as some books can be. Thank you everyone for helping me get this book into the public domain.

Colin, my ever loving husband, a huge thank you for being incredibly supportive, loyal and patient. I count myself blessed to have you in my life and love you and the life we share. Every day with you in it is a good day. Together, we care for any dog, cat, other animals and tree that comes our way.

David Lowry, my son, simply a beautiful person, who helped enormously with organising and arranging this book when it became simply too big. You had such patience on the subject and working with you was a pleasure. Your understanding, empathy and thoughtfulness are qualities you showed during the process, while you learnt more about what your mother talks about, quite a bit! I appreciate your time and commitment.

To my beautiful family; Kelly, Andrew, William and Katey, your understanding and respect for going along with us, to work with each of our dogs in the ways described within the following pages, has been mutually rewarding. Your love and empathy for all animals is part of who we are as a family and through the animals we have understood each other more! How wonderful life is, especially when you're in it. Thank you.

I owe so much to each dog and every rabbit, goat, pig, duck, chicken, cat, guinea-pig and chinchilla who have come into my life and taught me more than I thought possible. Each one of them has had a delightful character in their various ways and wonderful, unexpected relationships have formed. By living alongside one another they've taught me how to live with them peacefully; teaching me their language. Simply being able to observe beautiful creatures is such a gift and one of the most precious life offers. Thank you, which really only touches on the gratitude I feel.

Over the years my dogs and clients have been essential in guiding the course in learning, as each dog and client is unique, requiring different approaches and treatment. I've enjoyed working with you and your dogs to find paths through where both can feel at ease.

Also through working with clients some great friendships have formed, becoming dear lifelong friends. This job just keeps on giving, all thanks to the dogs – aren't they amazing?

Thank you to Sheila Harper and Winny Boerman who, amongst other things, are both applied zoopharmacognosy practitioners, for introducing us to self-selection as well as everything doggie.

Wow, what can I say about these two wonderful and caring people. You devote your lives to dogs of all shapes and sizes, helping their people too. My life certainly changed massively, bit by bit, when I met Sheila and attended one of her excellent canine behaviour courses many years ago. I couldn't wait to go back for more. And so I did. You both consider every dog and their needs above all else, which is a most refreshing way of looking at life: from the dogs' perspective. I've spent years searching for an approach that shows respect for dogs, then found it. Your approach is it!

Taken from Sheila's website because it says what they do:

Sheila Harper promotes high ethical standards working to build mutually respectful and responsive relationships between people and dogs. We are the leading education provider for dog trainers and behaviourists to learn about Real Life Skills. We also provide quality support for dog owners.

For Hagrid and I, almost whenever Sheila and Winny were needed you were available at the end of the phone, also squeezing extra visits in here and there too. Hagrid wasn't an easy dog to read and I appreciated your ongoing friendship, support and understanding.

Caroline Ingraham, the founder of Wild Health, and her colleague Martin Stubbs also came out to visit Hagrid at one point when he was seriously ill, giving up some of their precious time off!

Hayley Merron-Stevens, who listened to me talking about dogs so much, and then planted the seed to turn my writing about Hagrid into a book; and so it went. I value your gentleness, sensitivity and am so glad our paths crossed on life's interesting and varied journey. You're a beautiful person.

Chris Leeson's assistance with helping me to begin writing this book and setting the wheels in motion. Our time together was greatly appreciated. You understood me and what I wanted to say. Chris and I merged to develop Hagrid's life into words. Thank you.

Ann Lowe – ghostwriter, a warm and wonderful human being. Although this book was supposedly near completion when Ann stepped into the driving seat, it then took another turn complementing what was already there. Ann knew what I wanted to say and made it possible for us to explore other avenues together. It has been a wonderful adventure. You're such an inspirational lady and it's been a pleasure to have worked with you. Lyn Lowe, too. Thank you for your inspirational ideas contributing to the cover of the book.

Marilyn Aspinall who has been there as a friend and colleague throughout our travels with Hagrid, offering support and words of encouragement when life was so tough for all of us, especially him. We were able to work things out together and bounced ideas around. You are a true friend and supported us on our rollercoaster journey and are a true friend. I'll always be grateful for knowing you and for our friendship.

Jean Gough, another great friend and colleague. You helped Hagrid with trusting that humans aren't that scary after all. Having an understanding caring person around who would leave Hagrid to come round in his own time was something I'm really grateful for. That meant such a lot to Hagrid and us. Also, there was the part you played in the structure of this book, not to mention valid helpful suggestions and guidance. Thank you so much to you my lovely friend.

Miriam Krause, a friend and colleague who gives her time to help animals and people. Thank you for your input in this book, it's given us a valuable insight from a vet's point of view, one that some as pet carers rarely have access to. Miriam also attended Sheila Harper's courses to help her understand canine communication, which she applies in her work as a vet.

My sincere thanks to David Lowry, Pat Birkett, Marilyn Aspinall, Jean Gough, Ali Emm, Linda Maund and especially Jacqui and Jeremy Bassett for their continued, documented, concise critical feedback and eye for detail on reading this book. Every bit of advice has been welcomed, valid and carefully considered, making the finished book what it is today.

Thank you Jeremy for constructing some valid feedback, used to describe this book to others. Please see the website.

I'm also most appreciative to Stefan Dawson who, some years previously to designing and working on this book, worked for Colin in an office in our house. This was during some of Hagrid's life, so Stef knew Hagrid personally! And now Stef has designed this book, also helping with the later stages of editing. Your contribution has been invaluable. Working with you, Stef, has been an absolute pleasure and I hope the experience has inspired you to be involved in the making of many more books. Your work is thorough, you're conscientious and enthusiastic, have a good eye for detail and you're great at dealing with last minute changes.

My thanks to Hannah Sutton for giving your kind permission to include a cheeky photo of the delightful Nessa wallowing in a muddy puddle. What a dog!

And thank you Rachel Moore for kindly allowing me to use a photo of the adorable Shadow, exploring a fallen tree across a river.

Max appears with Pogo on a few photos, he's a beautiful sensitive soul: our neighbours Sandra and David Bailey kindly allow me to walk him now and then. You have a delightful dog, so thanks for allowing him to feature here.

Nicky, a lady I sometimes see while walking our dogs. She walks slowly for her dogs, who all have health issues, due to past neglect and bad treatment. Thank you for giving me permission to use the photos of your dogs with Pogo.

Thanks to Gerd Kohler again for donating one of his photos that I used for *Understanding the silent communication of dogs*. It's a lovely photo showing a play bow.

To everyone who listened to my requests to help Hagrid in situations he found difficult, we're most definitely grateful.

And to those who were able to come up with ideas to accommodate Hagrid's needs, easing the stress procedures can have on animals, giving him the best possible chance for healing, we were really thankful.

To everyone who has been involved in Hagrid's care and well-being and in the making of his book, I'm sincerely grateful, thank you.

I'd like you all to know that while I say 'thank you', they're not the words I am looking for to show the deep sense of gratitude and warmth I feel to everyone mentioned here. I find it quite overwhelming that you have contributed and given up your time to help in varied ways with this book. So while I 'thank you' it's not quite enough, but you'll know and understand that.

Foreword

Hagrid was not your average dog; he was a dog and a half, in more ways than one

By simply being, Hagrid taught me so much about himself. He was a dog that suffered physically and emotionally and having him come into my life nourished me in ways I didn't know were possible.

Every step of the way, it was Hagrid who did the teaching. Through him, I learned about myself, more about dogs in general and this hugely influenced my work as a behavioural advisor. I learned how to appreciate the small things in life.

How Hagrid did all of this is not entirely clear, however what matters is that I've made a commitment to share what I discovered along the way, so that others may benefit from the insights he provided.

In the beginning, we had no idea what we'd taken on. Everything about him was big; his presence, his paws, his head, his meals, his vet bills… His needs were big too in terms of his health issues and the energy required to help him with them.

In Hagrid, I was presented with almost every challenge that a dog carer can have. My job was to rise to those challenges, and to learn from Hagrid the ways that I could help him. It has been an incredibly interesting and rewarding journey, one that required commitment and willingness from not just me, but from my whole family as well.

What to expect from this book

The book started as therapy for me, by simply writing the thoughts I had the day after Hagrid was put to sleep. Like many in the same situation, I struggled to come to terms with the loss of my lovely dog in the beginning and took to writing as a way to help me process the emotions, hold onto and be reminded of the special memories of him. Then a good friend suggested I turn my thoughts into a book about Hagrid and what he had taught me, so that others could benefit too. And that's what happened.

My idea was that this book takes you on an adventure; one that will offer ideas and thoughts on how to explore creative solutions together with a dog, to the physical and emotional challenges they face. Throughout, I advocate slowing down, listening and letting a dog be the guide, rather than simply going with traditional advice. Considering all the options before making a choice for a dog opens up the possibility for greater communication and a deeper relationship.

Hagrid was a big dog, with an even bigger gift. I'll always be thankful to him for coming into our lives and will always feel him near me.

If all of us could be open enough to want to learn from our dogs, to listen to their communications, then I believe we would be able to build a much closer and more trusting relationship with them, and by doing so, open up the channels of communication when there are issues that need resolving. With a greater more empathetic relationship and by consciously working with dogs on decisions about their lives, we can help them so much more effectively and organically.

Through taking this approach, I, along with my family, were able to work with Hagrid through his health issues and because of this, he could open up, and trust me. And he gave so much back in return.

In this book, you'll find a few thoughts that may be useful in certain situations, but it doesn't contain cut and dried steps to follow. Every dog and every situation is unique and will benefit from a flexible rather than rigid approach.

Some areas addressed in the book are:

- How to develop trust between dog and carer.
- Barriers and boundaries.
- Respecting other animals.
- Teaching children and dogs to live together respectfully.
- Adjusting to new environments and experiences.
- Learning to use new behaviours.
- Exploring health treatments with which dogs are comfortable.
- Considering all elements of their lives when making decisions.

My hope is that the book will demonstrate, through Hagrid's story, that it is the way we treat a dog that leads to the most appropriate route of care. This means bringing a quality of awareness and openness to the relationship – a relationship of equals – so dogs can have their say. This builds trust and respect, in the same way that equality between humans does.

I'd like to share all of this with you because we really need to see that what we do, and the way we treat dogs, has implications for them. They are impacted a lot more by us than we may realise, in ways that we may have never noticed.

Through this book I want to continue all the lessons I learned from Hagrid, and to remember him by carrying on the legacy of the relationship we had.

This was his contribution to my life, both in the world of dog behaviour and in the outside world, so now, hopefully, this is my contribution to yours.

Even now as I close my eyes I can imagine exactly how it feels to stroke his knobbly chin and the feelings exchanged between us.

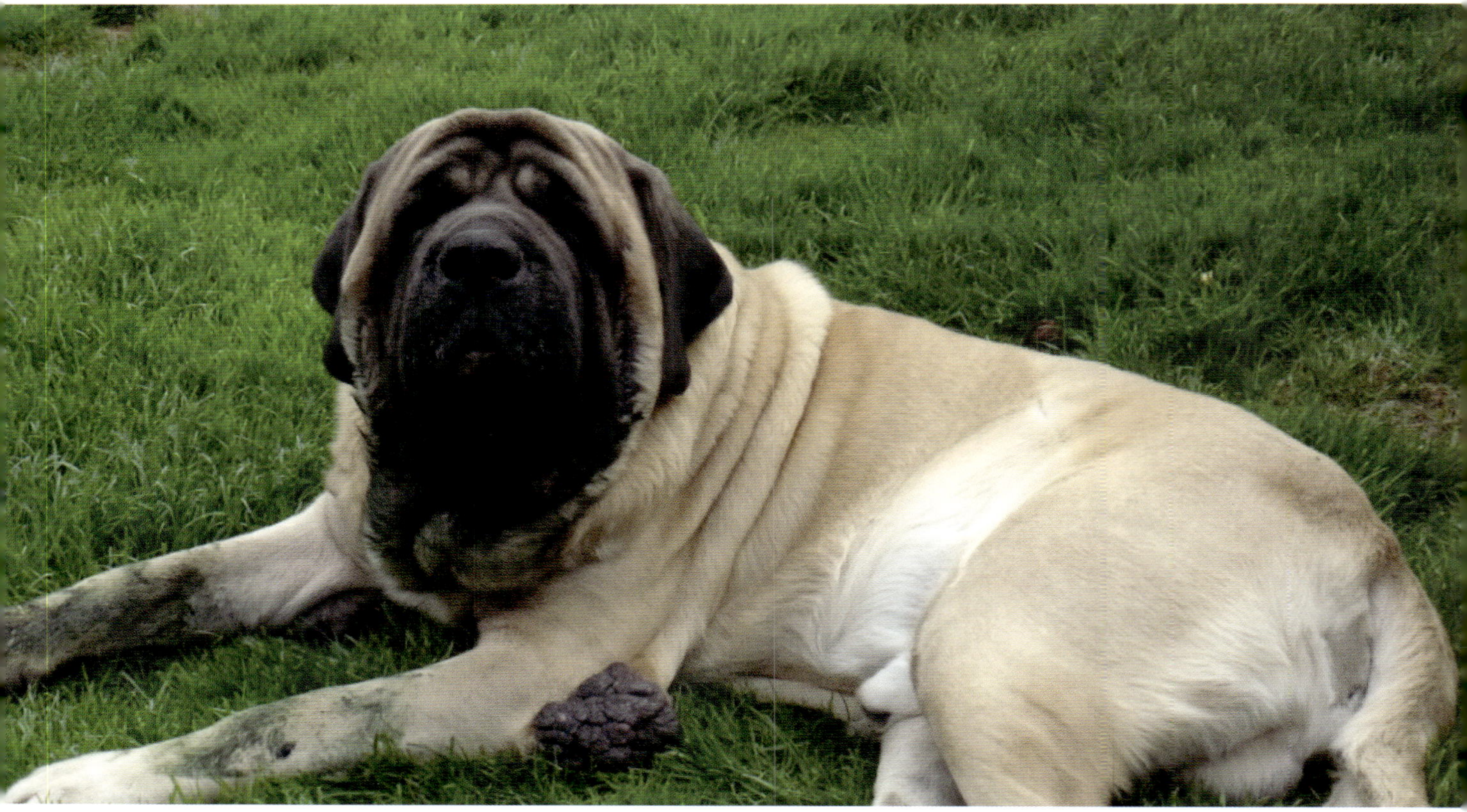

Thank you, Hagrid, for being you.

Chapter 1

Hagrid being put to sleep

At 4.30am on June 6th, the day after Hagrid was put to sleep, I decided to get up and go downstairs.

Up to this point I'd been lying in bed, trying desperately to sleep. But the bright morning sun shone through the curtains, and different thoughts and scenes from Hagrid's life were playing across my mind.

I reflected on what this beautiful dog had taught me – so many of life's simple lessons. These thoughts were difficult to push away, and as I tried to sleep, others would replace them. Two thoughts in particular kept me awake.

The first: sitting at the desk in my office that doubled as Hagrid's room, with him sleeping in his bed.

I remember how I used to be working then suddenly have this sense of being stared at. I'd look across and Hagrid would be gazing up at me with that gentle, melted soft look he had. It was a look of contentment and deep affection, and I was always compelled to stop and look back.

We'd just enjoy the time, looking at each other, giving one another attention. And sometimes he'd come over and lay his heavy head on my lap while I slowly – that is, at his pace – stroked his head and neck.

This was just a great, simple time for us to deepen our bond.

The second thought came as I lay there, aware of my breath and how it felt when it touched my arm. This reminded me of the vivid feeling I'd experienced while sitting with Hagrid's head in my arms as he lay on the floor in the kitchen the previous day. I'd wait to feel his next breath and was struck by how slow his breathing was.

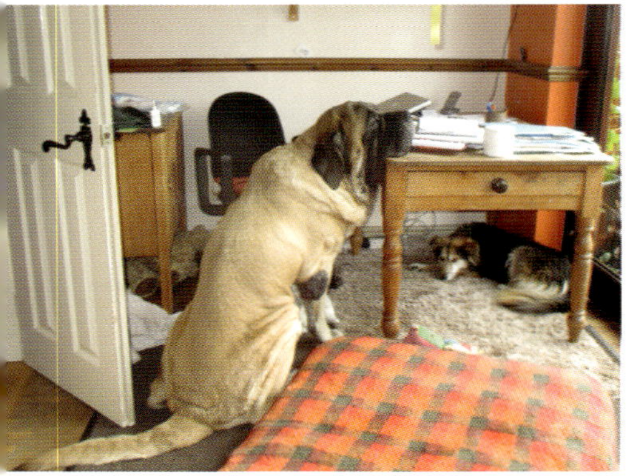

A usual scene in my office as I worked. Pogo and Hagrid close by. Hagrid would often come and lay his head on my desk or lap.

Hagrid's breath had always been so slow, with long pauses in between. I have fond memories of waiting for him to breathe out and wondering how deep that air must've gone into his body. In fact, everything about Hagrid was slow, but if you were prepared to wait, as I was, it all happened in good time.

Whilst he'd been ill, it had taken him much more time to do pretty much anything. In fact, life for us all had become even slower. Hagrid needed longer to process information; although when he was given the time, he'd make good decisions and was clear in what he needed or wanted (and how he was going to do it!). And I'd learned – as far as possible – to adjust with him and suppress my anxiety or my need to move faster.

So, on the morning of 6th June as I left my bed, with a mind full of memories, I took the decision to go into the kitchen via the lounge. This is because, on that particular day, it was the first morning without my beloved Hagrid. On any other day, I'd have walked into the kitchen and seen Hagrid, my dog, my soul mate: a full thirteen stones of English Mastiff, lying sprawled out somewhere on the stone tiled floor. He loved the coolness of those floor tiles.

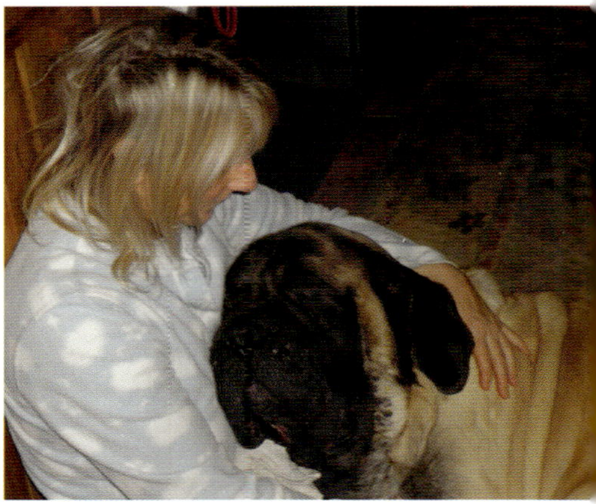

Most mornings were spent like this while we slowly awoke. Just a few minutes with each dog in the mornings is a great start to the day. This is how it was on the morning before the day he was put to sleep. Oh, I miss you Hagrid.

This was an extremely painful time for me.

Hagrid was put to sleep on June 5th, in the afternoon at 3.15pm.

In the last week or so, as a product of the possible brain tumour, Hagrid had been unable to get himself up without help and support, and now he was losing the strength in his back legs. Placing his feet on the ground took time, even with my help, and was so much mental effort for him. It was another backwards step and I felt I couldn't let him go through any further trauma.

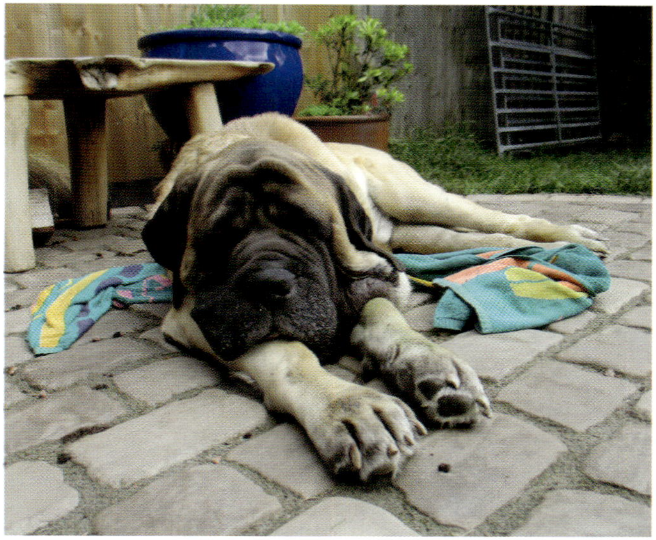

Resting on the patio three days before he was put to sleep. The towel was used to help him get about. At first Hagrid and I could manage in the garden, now it required two of us to help him outside.

On the morning of the day he was put to sleep, it was as though he'd given up, and his dignity had gone.

Hagrid didn't like the fact that he had to be helped up and guided with each footstep, even though we waited together until he was ready to make the next move. Before the back legs lost strength, he'd been struggling to get his front legs to work effectively and now all four legs were affected.

Helping Hagrid as I had done was what I wanted to do, but something was telling me that this wasn't fair, as he couldn't get outside unaided. Moreover, I could no longer help him to get up on my own.

This was the end, despite him still eating and drinking well. There was no problem in him being able to communicate his need to go outside. The harsh truth was that the time had come to assist him in his final moments.

Hagrid's favourite vet, Graham, came out for a home visit. They first met about two weeks after Hagrid started to live with us. Graham had always been respectful of him; maybe both had shown fear at first, as Hagrid didn't easily trust people. Up until that point, it had been a quiet and calm, hot early June day. Heat had always made Hagrid seem subdued. For much of the day, he'd been lying on the kitchen floor as he'd done for the whole night. His habits and patterns had changed; he'd stopped lying in his bed because it became too difficult to negotiate, mentally and physically.

The house was purposely peaceful and calm, with healing animal music playing quietly. The pace was slow, which Hagrid enjoyed. We'd often be together like this, which was quality time for us. It was a bittersweet feeling for me and I felt unsettled, finding it hard to really be with him. I so deeply wanted to be there with him emotionally, spiritually, but the thought of losing him later was unbearable. Part of me was connected to him as we sat on the floor but I couldn't tell how he felt. I wanted to have the old Hagrid back and at the same time knew it was unfair to keep him alive in his condition.

When I reflect on the account of Hagrid's last day and how it's described in this book, I feel that there's a slight disconnect with my description and the reality. I've tried so hard to capture the events as they happened, but all the same it sounds as though the house was calm, and I spent the whole day with Hagrid. It was, and I did, but was doing jobs in between. I cried a lot. I found it hard to settle. There were also moments when I could 'be' with Hagrid, and moments when I couldn't; although I wanted to, it was painful to be with him. Doing what was best for Hagrid is what I wanted, yet it was so hard not to get emotional. I tried as much as possible to hide that from him.

But when I look back on that day, what really matters is that, thankfully, the needle went into his vein easily and he felt no more suffering. And so, this was the day when Hagrid left us. He was at home with everyone who loved him and as I held him, I felt the energy drain from his body. Then I knew he was gone.

Anyone who has lost a beloved pet will know there are many ways in which their presence is missed. Some of the ways are expected, but many are not. Losing an animal can affect us deeply and the feeling of loss can be triggered by almost anything.

I so missed Hagrid. His whole lovely presence. His heavy head on my lap, his wagging tail when I came in or if he heard me, even the sound of him breathing - a gentle, consistent noise in the house. The calming times we had together, too: being interrupted because he wanted fuss, or his over-excitement to see me if I'd been out for more than a few hours. One physical lasting memory, soon to fade, that I really didn't want to lose was being trodden on and getting bruises on my feet!

I missed wiping Hagrid's face several times a day after food and often cleaning his eyes, his ears, his slobber, and needing to have towels in every room. I'd have given anything for all of these experiences again. The smelly ears and the deep ache I felt when he rolled around the floor with itchy ears as I tried ways to ease his pain; his smell, mainly due to his skin condition; wiping the patio windows where he'd pushed his face against them; bumping into furniture or people; covers on furniture and the floor; even the ramp we used for Hagrid to get him in and out of the van towards the end of his life.

Then there were the walks, and his slow, thorough investigation of the environment, sitting down, taking in the day and all nature had to offer. I loved everything that came with Hagrid, especially the inspirational times. All the cooking involved with his food, the preparation of veggies, coconuts and carrots; the way he asked for the vegetables; all the food he needed, cooking fish and lentils in bulk; water bowl spillages and drinking buckets; and then there was barking to come and go from the house; closing and opening doors and gates.

There was always plenty to remind me of him. Even just being in the way and having to step over such a big dog or waiting for him to move before going past. What touched me most was the process of his slow thoughtfulness. His way.

I loved all that came with Hagrid.

Above all, I was left with memories, the most powerful of which – and the one that overwhelmed me with grief – was experiencing daily life sitting at the computer in my office/Hagrid's bedroom, and having a sense of being stared at. The thought of his gorgeous face made me melt into tears.

CHAPTER 2

An introduction to the other dogs in this book

While much of the writing focuses on Hagrid's life, there are times when it's been valuable to draw on the experiences of other dogs that I've cared for. I talk about and have used photographs of them to help illustrate various points, so it's helpful to understand who they are.

Throughout this book you'll be introduced to my wonderful, loving, supportive and patient husband, Colin, and you'll also meet Jaffa and Pogo, who have both shared their lives with us at different times, as well as Henry and Kaos; the latter was with us just before Hagrid.

At the time of writing this book, Kuzu and Daisy have joined our household and have been particularly helpful in illustrating how to introduce a dog to a new home plus the boundaries that need to be in place between them and our other animals.

The next few pages are dedicated to photos of these other four-legged companions with whom I've shared my life.

Jaffa, a Cavalier King Charles Spaniel

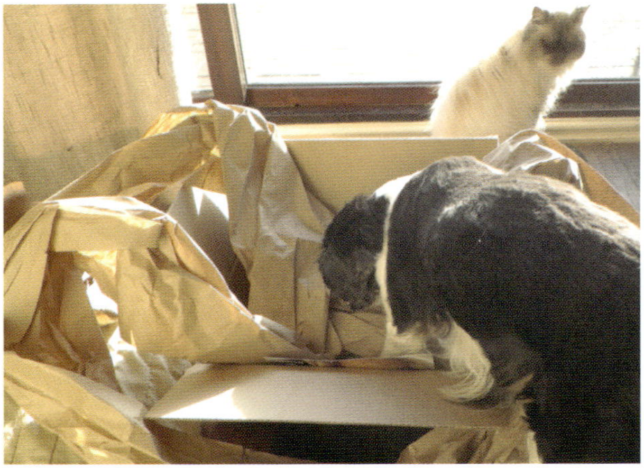

Jaffa exploring a box.

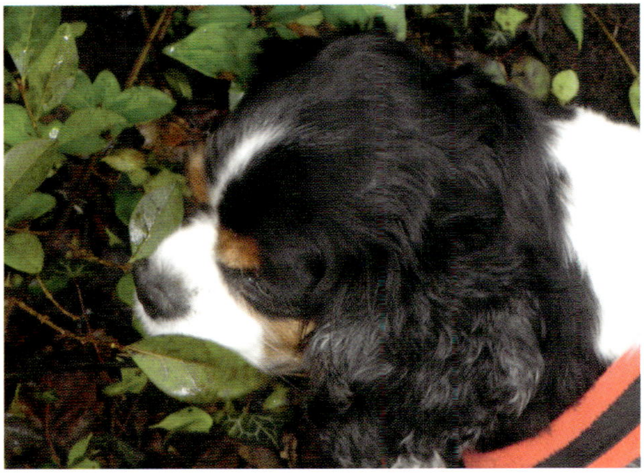

Doing what she loved: being inquisitive.

Henry, a Clumber Spaniel

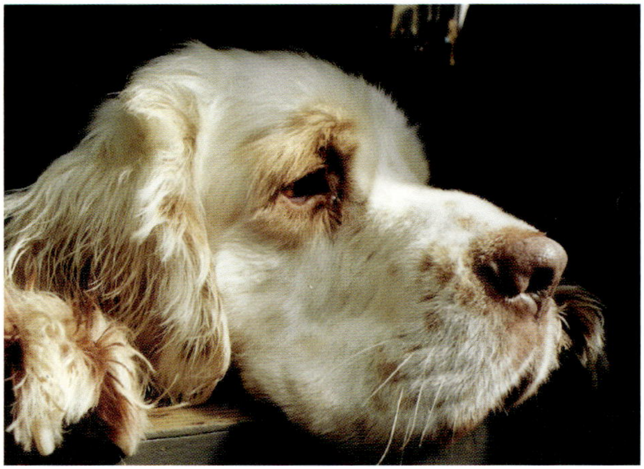

Henry, enjoying happier times.

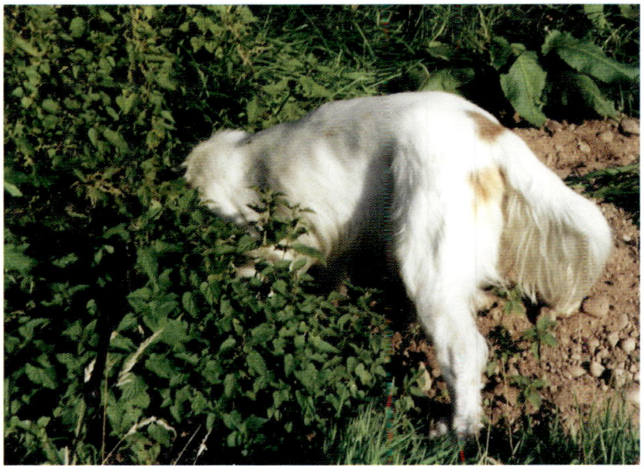

Exploring holes in the earth was a favourite pastime for Henry.

Kaos, an English Mastiff

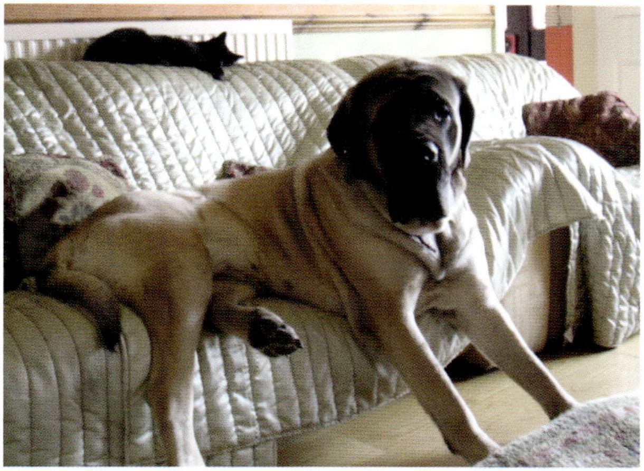

Here's Kaos relaxing...

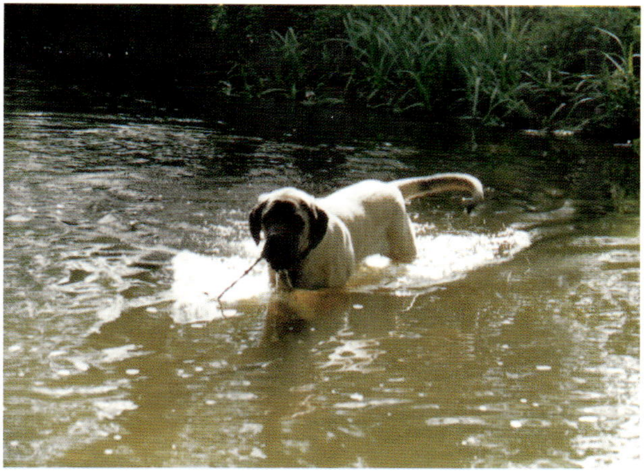

... and then finding adventure in the river.

Pogo, a Samoyed crossed with other breeds

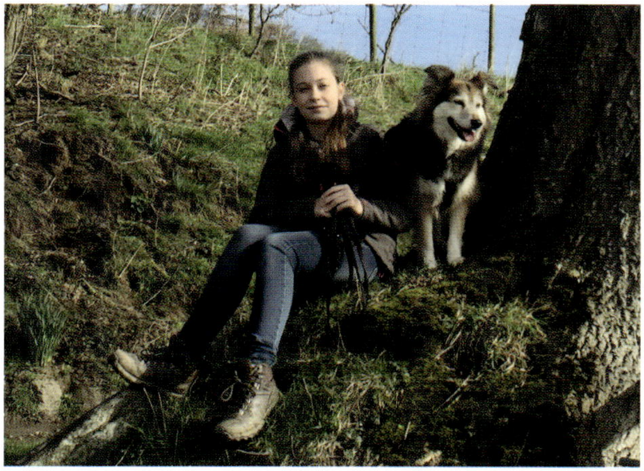

Pogo taking an interest in all that's going on.

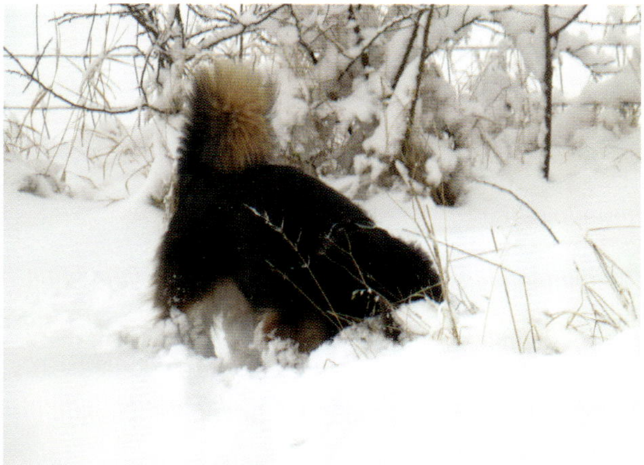

Pogo in her element, finding what's beneath the snow.

Kuzu, an Anatolian Shepherd crossed with Mastiff

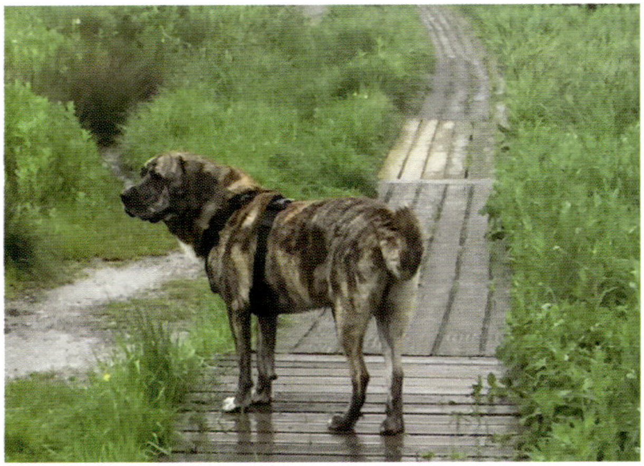

This is Kuzu who joined us late in 2015.

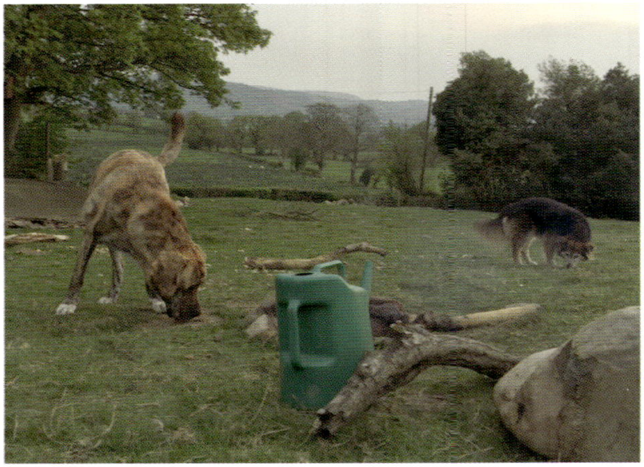

Together Pogo and Kuzu investigate goings on in a field.

Daisy, a Staffordshire Bull terrier cross

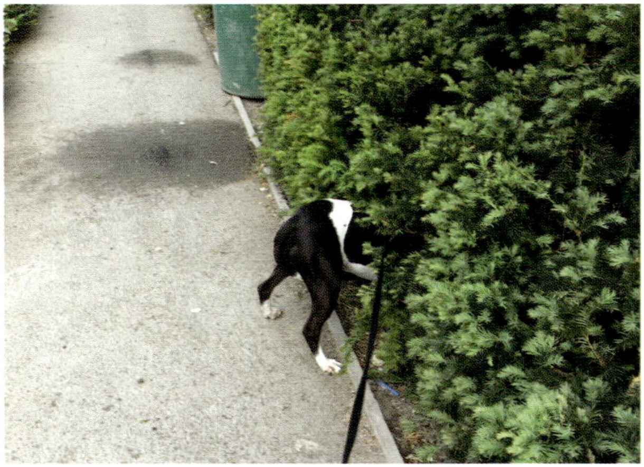

Daisy using her efficient nose to track down a morsel of food.

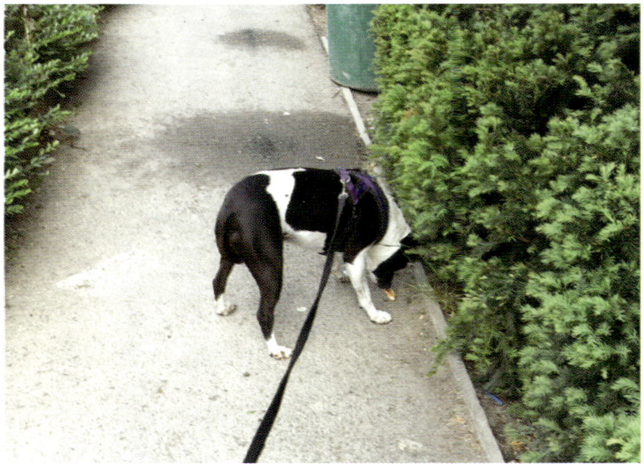

Found it! One of Daisy's favourite walks where people picnic. She likes to explore the bushes for leftovers.

CHAPTER 3

Introducing Hagrid to our home

The first few weeks of having a new dog

Every dog comes from somewhere: whether that's a reputable breeder or rescue centre, someone else's home, or sadly from a puppy farm. Of course, the place they're taken to is going to be very different from what they'd been used to.

No two environments, people or routines are identical, and dogs need plenty of time to observe and settle before they can be a part of what's going on.

When meeting a new dog, it's not entirely possible to know what their previous life was like, their perception and how they're going to behave in a new situation. The age of the dog can also be a factor. Puppies require different handling to middle-aged or older dogs, and those who have been mistreated or are ill need the right systems in place to ensure they feel safe and well.

This isn't to say that puppies are all the same. Some have baggage passed on from their parents' genes and they've been brought up in different places. Other conditions from the mother can play a part too, in terms of the environment, her life experiences and perceptions, as well as her emotional and physical condition while the unborn pups were developing. How she brings them up has an impact on each one.

Puppies will be affected in their individual way. The age that they leave their mother and the nature of the separation all comes into the equation. Then the new environment they find themselves in, and the surrounding area also play a part.

Throughout these stages, people are invariably involved with their own set of circumstances, which will have a bearing on all of the dogs. While we can influence puppies in some ways, nothing is guaranteed with regard to their treatment and individual temperament.

I will use analogies with children throughout this book because there are good parallels. Bringing a new dog home is like bringing a child home; everyone needs time to adjust, especially the child. The good news is that parents can do a lot to make things easier, and the same goes for anyone who cares for dogs.

> Every re-homed dog needs time to adapt to new surroundings and have things introduced slowly.

Hagrid needed lots of time to get used to us, our routines and how we responded to everyday situations, and as with any new dog in our household, we managed his introduction to our home and our other animals with care and attention.

The settling-in period is usually much longer than most people realise. It can be months and often longer depending on different factors. I feel most dogs would do much better if they were given this luxury and maybe more would stay and settle in their homes if their early weeks and months were handled sensitively. This includes the introductions to other members of the family, particularly children, other animals, new places and even exercise.

It's relatively common for people to take on a re-homed dog then return it shortly after, sometimes as little as a week or two. When asked what's happened in that time, the underlying reason is often that the dog was expected to endure too much and exposed to doing things way too soon.

Unintentionally, children can be a major factor in this, as they might not be used to dealing with dogs. The children may be not have been given clear boundaries, be overly excitable, they might pull the dog's tail, hug, sit on them or interact with them in a way that's uncomfortable. A dog who reacts is then considered to be difficult or dangerous and taken back.

This yo-yo-ing back and forth from home to rescue is so destructive and damaging for dogs on an emotional and physical level. The experience affects some so dramatically that it results in their loss of life.

Of course, I see why people usually want to be kind to a rescue dog and it's entirely possible to do this, though it may not be what we *think* they need. There can be a tendency to overwhelm dogs in the first few days and weeks, exposing them to all types of things that they aren't ready for yet. Some dogs appear to be dealing with everything until around the second week or so, then unwanted behaviours begin to emerge. This could be because the dog had been worried about showing their emotions early on.

As time goes by, however, a dog may feel unable to hold these emotions in any longer and express them by doing things we may deem unacceptable. Roughly from ten months to two years old (sometimes described as the teenage time for dogs) it's common for quite a few to be discarded from their homes and sent off to a new home or rescue centre. It can be a challenging time for dogs and their carers.

That means something isn't suiting the dog and it's their way of letting us know, and the longer it's left, the more frustration builds.

Being prepared to accept that things might not run smoothly when taking on a rescue dog (any dog) can help take the pressure off both carer and dog. Accepting and working with them if problems arise can be helpful and avoid clashes, meaning that problems are likely to dissipate far sooner than if they were met with conflict. Dogs may often be destructive, soil their surroundings, try to escape, steal things, jump up, bark, and be wary of people and other dogs. They are likely to whine and howl, sometimes for a few weeks. Puppies too are quite likely to do any or all of the above.

It's how we deal with things that determines what happens next.

Initial support

Dogs frequently require *lots* of time to get used to their immediate surroundings before being exposed to people, other dogs, animals, long walks, traffic and so on. They also need outlets for their behaviour, of course within flexible and appropriate boundaries, just as we do. Trying to accommodate those emotions and giving the dog time to settle fully is key to success. Later, probably much later, depending on the dog, it will be possible to slowly expose them to a wider environment.

That's what worked for us with Hagrid and all our dogs; supporting him on a long lead (five metres) while in the garden, and allowing him to explore in his own time. We did this for a few weeks until he was definitely confident and settled, without racing around or reacting to things he smelt, heard or saw. His needs were being met because I was there supporting him if he felt worried by anything in the new environment, as quite a few dogs do. He had the time and space to do what he needed within thought-out boundaries. If he got overexcited at any time we took a step back.

People often say to me about their dog, "He'd been let out and was outside for ages, then came in the house and went to the toilet." There can be many reasons for this and a common one is because the dog is feeling insecure in some way.

If he feels safe and is supported outside, this can be ruled out as a contributing factor to the behaviour. I've found that a few months of hard work in the beginning pays dividends in the long run and is so worth the time and effort.

Having the opportunity for plenty of sleep and rest during the day as well as night (16-18 hours for an adult and 18+ for puppies) will go a long way in settling a newcomer.

At this time, dogs are also learning about their new family, and by doing these things for them in a gentle way, the bond can become a good, solid one from the start. Learning that they can rely on their carer will help them feel secure.

The way the lead is used is important and can result in a dog reacting to something or not. Leads are discussed in more detail later, in the chapter on Walks.

We influence dogs so much by the way they're handled. A great way to communicate relaxed trust is to use the lead gently, lightly and sensitively, a little like the way it feels to hold hands. This enables a supportive and safe connection. When the lead trails after the dog there's a sense of detachment and of being separate. Dogs are often left flailing at the end of a long lead.

Some dogs can have a short attention span, often due to what's happened to them previously. Puppies too have short attention spans. After a few weeks, when the dog seems more settled, used to the routine, and generally more grounded, the lead can be on while he's in the garden, then casually unclipped maybe for a few seconds.

During these times with Hagrid, I was mindful to see what he did. If he pottered around as he sniffed, this was a sign that he was settling into the new routine and beginning to feel at ease. The lead was re-attached after a very short time while I took him back inside again, and this was a positive experience that I built on.

It was worth repeating these early stages because when we learn or teach, there is a pressure to always get better, which produces specific expectations. If the boundaries/limitations and barriers had been suddenly removed because it seemed Hagrid was fine now, he was likely to feel lost without knowing what was expected. That's why it needed to be a slow process, occasionally retracing steps. It ensured the best possible chance of success for both of us.

When doing anything with a new dog it's beneficial to have a similar process: a short experience, aiming for success and then returning to the safety of familiarity. Having these brief exposures to things gave Hagrid the chance to learn and develop his skills for dealing with life. By avoiding 'too much, too soon', we established boundaries, and then gradually opened them up slowly. Being over excitable, as might happen in a new situation, can be a sign of not coping well.

Think about when we were babies: we needed security and love, and if this were done well, we were able to grow, open up and explore the world. We couldn't do this quite as well if we came from a fearful place.

Timing

Everything in life needs time. We only need to look at the seasons and how they work to make way for new things. Taking time is important.

Interestingly, as I was writing this chapter, we lost our internet connection. I was impatient, trying to get it back up, but it needed time to reboot. I left it alone, and it fixed itself. That made me think. I knew to give the Wi-Fi time, but I think a lot of us are like this and don't allow ourselves and our animals time in the same way. If we could do this, we might see that some things get fixed by pretty much just leaving them alone! Less is more in many respects. I appreciate that giving ourselves or our dogs time isn't always easy, but it is enlightening if we allow ourselves to do so. Somehow, it also relieves pressure.

Hagrid was a dog that needed time and then some! Everything he did was slow. I'd realised this, in the way that we all need different speeds. The countryside has a different pace to the city, and everyone will have a different internal speed depending on many factors, such as where we were brought up and the family who raised us.

Pogo's speed was the opposite of Hagrid's when she came to live with us. However, her speed was caused by something given to her by human involvement; a dog wouldn't naturally be as 'wired' as she was.

With lots of time and by utilising some of the suggestions in this book that were relevant to her, she has become a really sensible dog who no longer jumps over dog gates, stable doors, and right up onto work surfaces!

As an aside, it's really interesting how she uses her new skills to help other dogs. The teaching begins by her moving slowly and taking her time, while she gently observes the other dog. They see her slowly walking along; stopping to sniff at this and that in her environment and are almost always calmed by her slowness. She does this on purpose.

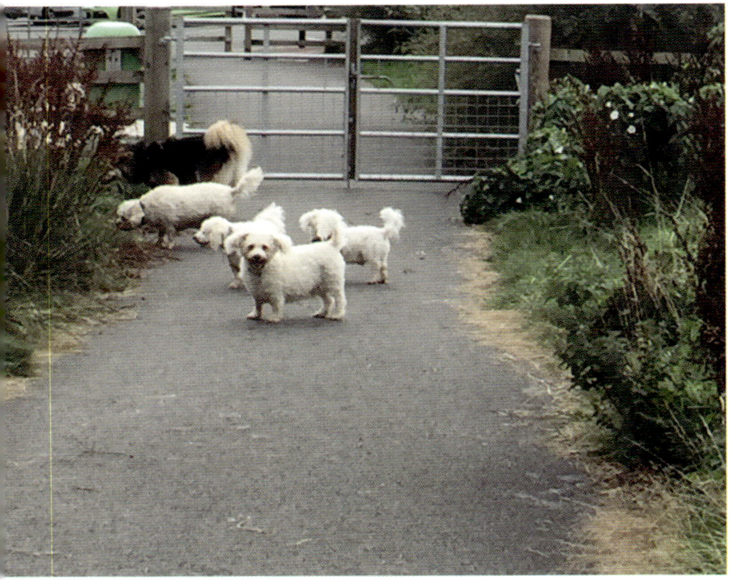

I love to see the influence she has on other animals: it's quite amazing. This is a result of using boundaries, limitations and barriers that were appropriate and fluid as she developed.

It was important to Pogo for me to accept her for the dog she was, not the dog I'd imagined she'd be.

While Pogo can manage well off-lead in many situations, we still use boundaries for her so she can feel safe and so she isn't subjected to too much emotional pressure. She appreciates this and at times can show relief when her lead is clipped back on. After all, we all need regular breaks.

Pogo had been gradually introduced to these dogs over time while on lead and so was comfortable to meet and potter about with them for a couple of minutes before we carried on with our walk.

Some parents can be in a rush to teach their children to walk, talk and read. Perhaps there's a sense of pride that their child is 'advanced', although I'm not sure if the rushing and the pressure are in the ultimate interests of the child. The same applies to our dogs. There is often pressure on dog carers for their dogs to behave, particularly in front of other people, whatever the age or background of the dog. But in a lot of cases, this pressure can have the opposite effect.

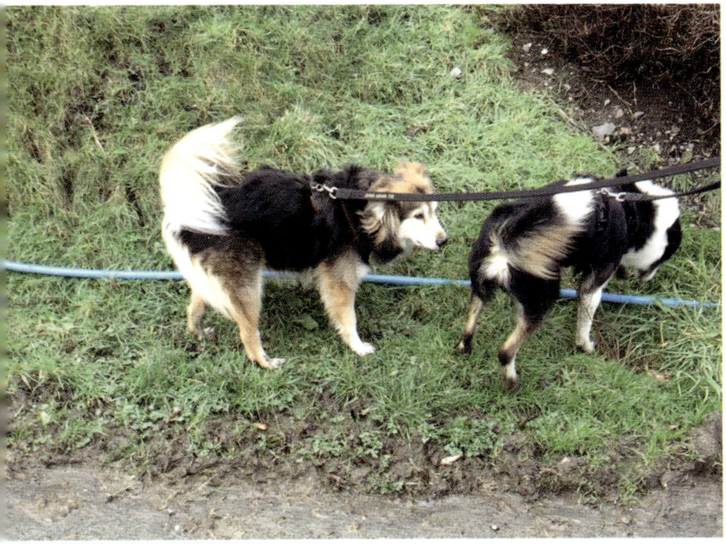

Max and Pogo had gradually become acquainted and regularly shared short walks. Here, Pogo gives Max some space and time to sniff.

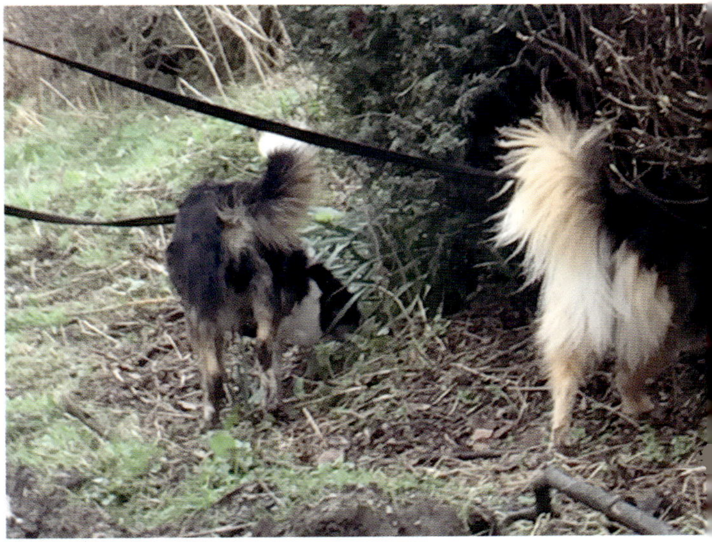

Max was rather excited at the start of his walk, so Pogo was mindful and waited until a little later before joining up with him to share the experience.

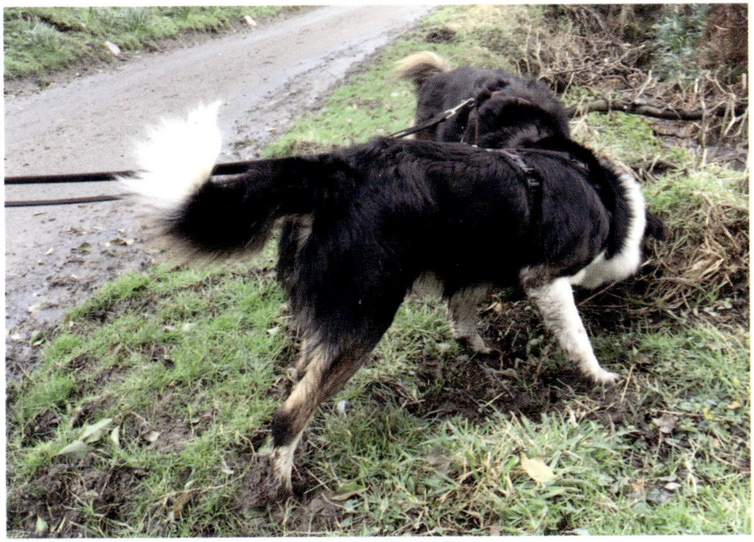

Some dogs can share in this way and it's possible for them to learn this and taking their time gives them the opportunity to think.

What we learnt

- Using a long, static lead when introducing our dogs to the garden or outside area helped them feel secure and safe. Waiting with them and following them as they explored, then doing this for a few weeks, sometimes longer, helped their confidence.

- Putting in the work early on gave the dogs a solid base to build upon. I can't emphasise this enough.

- Our dogs did well with limited space in the house to begin with, then we slowly expanded their environment as they settled and adapted.

- I made sure each dog had the opportunity for 18 hours or more sleep and quality rest each day.

- Having patience and understanding that Hagrid and Pogo were likely to be anxious and have difficulty settling in. Hagrid wanted to be left alone with someone nearby, whereas Pogo needed less space and someone close at hand for support.

- Colin and I were prepared to sleep near the new dogs for the first few nights while they adapted to their surroundings. When Kuzu came to our house, I slept on the kitchen floor with a dog gate between us so he could settle. He'd shown he was a little unsure of people. Hagrid was different; he also didn't trust people, but during the night he came to sniff me as I lay on the settee and then went into a smaller adjoining room, which became his bedroom. All of the dogs needed to go out into the garden during the night while settling in.

- If any of them needed to be walked, the walks were initially very short, usually a matter of minutes and in a quiet place, at a quiet time on a long line.

Introducing dogs to each other

By taking the time to introduce the dogs already in our house, the new dog settled better than if the introduction had been rushed or done without care and attention. If the experience is less stressful then they can get to know each other gradually, at their own pace.

An existing dog in the home will likely choose to explore a new dog when they're relaxed, so it was important to create the conditions for this natural style of learning to take place.

That's what happened in the past with Jaffa and Hagrid, Pogo and Hagrid, and (here) for Pogo and Kuzu. Using a dog gate ensured that they were separate and treated as individuals, especially for the settling-in period. This helped the existing dog as often it's hard for them when a new dog shares their resources. Both of them benefitted from having their own space and could see each other if they chose to, but were able to be away from the other as and when they wanted.

Kuzu and Pogo were now more or less comfortable with each other for short periods. He was a rescue dog, just as Pogo was. Pogo liked him, but to maintain a positive relationship they needed our help and guidance for a long time, for them to feel totally at ease with one another. This meant time together and time apart. Kuzu was a young, exuberant dog, so Pogo was happy to have regular breaks from him daily. It can be tiring for a dog to have the responsibility of an exuberant young dog, without breaks. Each dog required a barrier for large parts of the day and night, coming together at quiet times of the day.

If we hadn't taken these steps, Kuzu would have carried on using the behaviours that he'd known before: heavily pawing other dogs with both front paws, invading their space and bouncing around.

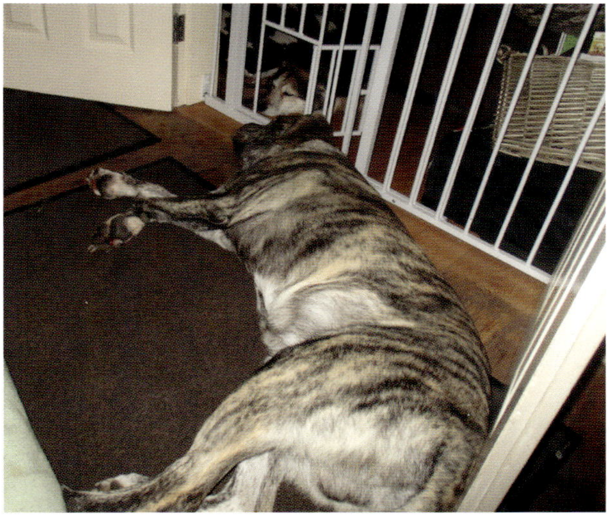

So this is Kuzu, not Hagrid, and I've used this photo because it's clear how after just a week, Pogo has chosen to go closer to Kuzu while he's sleeping, when she felt it was safe. It's good for someone to be in the room with each dog to begin with until both dogs are okay being in a room by themselves.

This was in fact a good way to keep other dogs away! It was quite effective and this may have been why he used it. But he never uses his paws in this way now; given time, he's largely a thinking dog rather than a reacting dog.

When Hagrid came to our house, Jaffa already lived with us. She actually chose Hagrid as the Mastiff to come and live with us. We'd seen other adult Mastiffs that required a home, but he was the one she felt more at ease with and wanted to meet.

They had a short, on-lead walk in a field together with a great distance between them. Jaffa followed him, and she and I were able to walk parallel with him at some points during the walks. This took place a couple of times before Hagrid came back to our house, and both were accepting of each other as they met. No fuss was made, it was a case of acknowledging each other, then moving on.

Both were treated as individuals so that Jaffa still felt safe and had our attention, giving her the routine she was accustomed to while gradually introducing Hagrid, and he could get used to her and us from a safe distance. They genuinely liked one another so it wasn't too long before they were around each other more and more.

For Hagrid and Pogo it took quite a bit longer. Prior to Pogo coming home with us for the first time, we took them both for a walk individually; I took Hagrid, and Colin took Pogo. We allowed for a brief meeting at a gate and then went in separate directions.

After this initial meeting, we then went into the house separately and took them to different areas that we'd designated as theirs. Before the walk it had been useful to spend time to set up the space in the house and garden so that they could be apart. A few weeks later once they were familiar with each other we could then bring them together at quieter times, if Hagrid was asleep for example. We'd open the gate that separated them and casually leave it open, not making an announcement or a big deal of it.

If Hagrid woke up and wanted to explore, Pogo found that difficult to deal with initially. Of course, the dogs sometimes noticed that the gate was open in their snoozy state but by that time it wasn't a big deal. They spot most things even if we think they are sleeping.

When dogs are deeply asleep, that's when they are totally relaxed and feel safe. It was a long time before Pogo could do that; the process took some time for her to feel safe around Hagrid due to him being clumsy. Being aware of what was going on and walking between them, to keep them apart, when we could see Pogo might struggle with him being close, helped both and taught him what was acceptable.

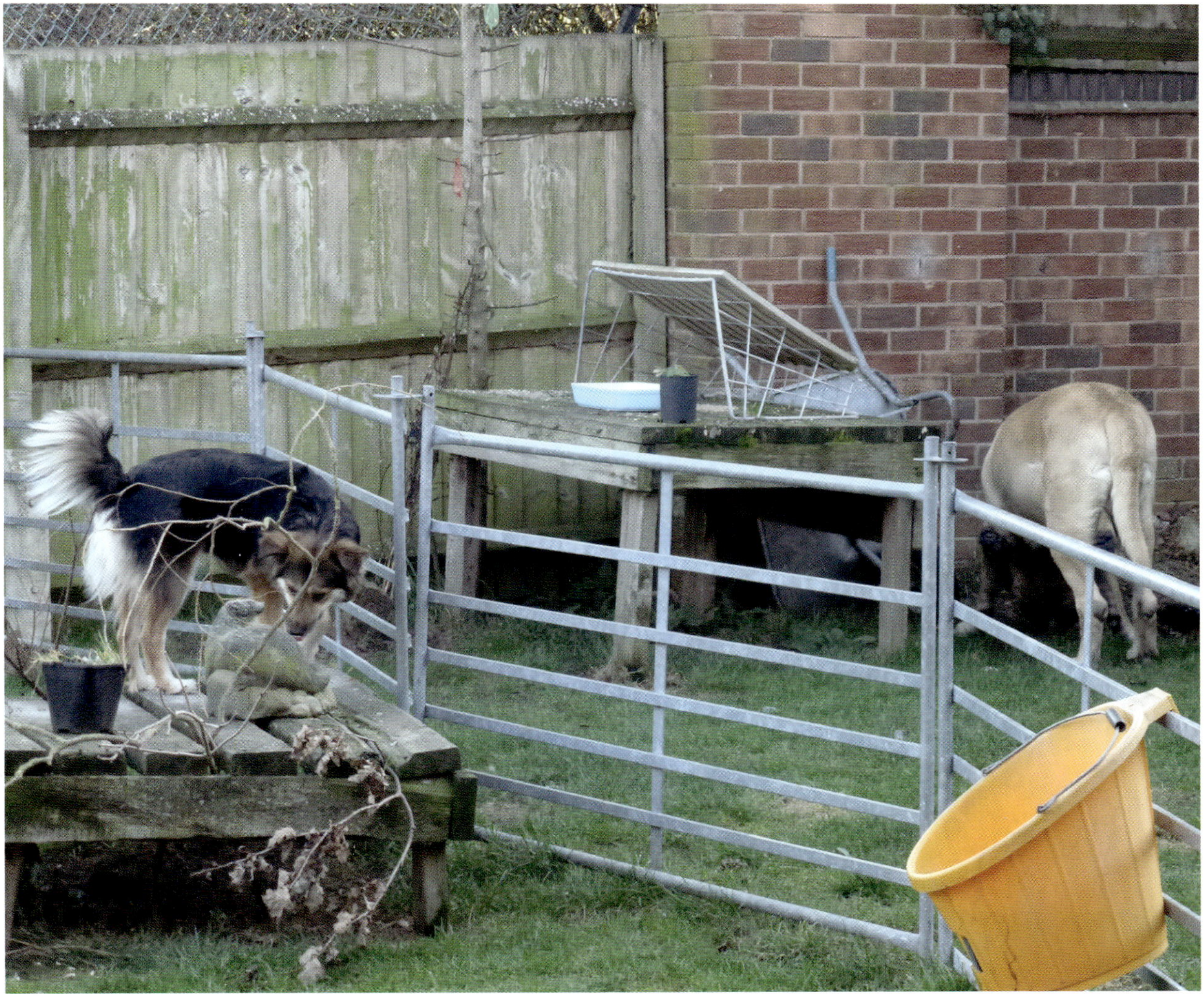

For the first few weeks Pogo was on lead every time she went outside in the garden and in the house too. The space that she occupied in the garage was somewhere she could be off lead. As well as having barriers outside, we put up dog gates at various doorways inside the house, helping both slowly and safely adapt and get to know one another in their own time. They can decide how close to be and when to move nearer to the other dog, but each one needs to feel safe from behind the gates before coming together.

If one of them went through the gate, we'd observe and then separate them whenever it was appropriate, by closing the gate. It's best to finish on success. One dog would follow, or could casually be distracted, then the gate would be closed again.

It took a while, but over time we were able to let them be together more frequently and for more extended periods, walking in between them if needed. This is another way to give them space and change the intensity. When visitors came and went, after food and at other exciting times, they were kept apart. Dogs generally find these times more difficult.

It does depend on the individual dogs though; on their temperament, background and communication they show. In general we found it better to take it easy at first even when it seemed to be going well, leaving things on a positive note.

All dogs will have their preferred signs, it's a matter of learning to recognise them and separating them before things escalate.

Being split up when low-level signals appear will help both dogs and positively enhance any developing relationship. When there's consistency with the process they'll gradually learn to make sensible choices for themselves, requiring far less intervention.

Some signs to separate the dogs included:

- Agitation from either dog when they're moving around quickly.
- Slowing down or being still.
- Play bows (see photo) - sometimes mean a dog is uncomfortable, showing appeasement and not coping well. This is what Pogo did.
- Standing by a door, even momentarily, can indicate their need to get out of the situation.
- Looking for help.

Feeding separately and out of sight of one another, with a barrier keeping the dogs apart, was something we did and still do. There can be tension when they are fed together even if it isn't always obvious. I can feel it sometimes when I watch our dogs, even with a see-through barrier. Just the presence of a dog can make another feel slightly uncomfortable. Are they going to try and steal their food?

By feeding them separately, with a solid, physical barrier they don't feel threat or pressure to bolt food down or not eat, so have time to enjoy it.

We also applied the same ideas to their sleeping arrangements. Some dogs genuinely like sleeping with one another, but bear in mind that not all will get up and move away if they're uncomfortable sleeping in close proximity. Observing this is one key to understanding whether dogs living together really get on.

Giving them separate sleeping places could be an excellent idea for all dogs so that they can make a choice about where to be. It may be possible to subtly video or take photos to look properly at the scene. At times, playing video footage back at a slow speed helped us to consider their communication and body language. However, I've found that videoing dogs can change their behaviour and they may not actually be comfortable with it, so care needs to be taken. I've learned that a discreet approach works best.

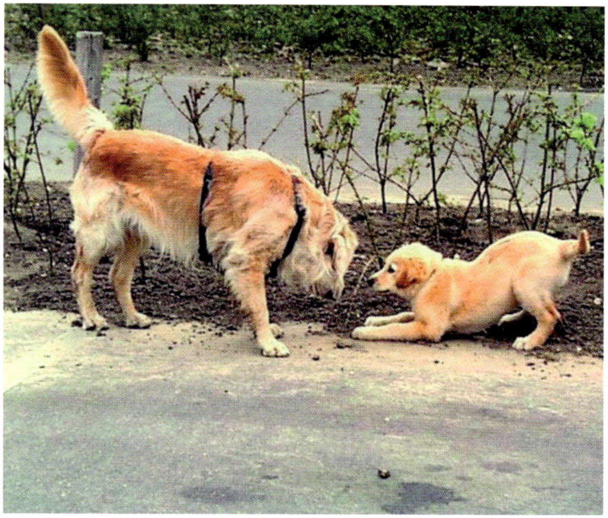

The puppy is giving the adult dog a signal, known as a 'play bow' because often a dog will use this toward another to initiate play. From observation it is also used to convey other messages, sometimes when a dog is fearful, intending no harm.

(Thanks to Gerd Kohler for this photo)

CHAPTER 4

Relationship with other animals

Inside the home – Hagrid's relationship with our other dog, Jaffa

I was aware that Jaffa needed looking after while Hagrid eased into his new life with us. Although Jaffa liked Hagrid, she still needed protecting, especially due to their size difference; she was a small King Charles Cavalier.

Both physical and emotional boundaries were put in place. These included dog gates to protect their personal space, rearranging furniture to better suit both of them, putting them on leads, and using our body language.

For several weeks/months, the two dogs were never left alone together without someone in the room; that way we could intervene if needed, before either became uncomfortable. Jaffa had more access to the house than Hagrid as she was able to get upstairs whereas he never attempted to go up there; later we found out he couldn't. We didn't know Hagrid; this would take some months. I did, however begin to notice that he was sometimes quite clumsy.

Over the years, I've shared my life with many dogs and know how long it can take them to fully settle in, sometimes up to a year and even longer, depending on a variety of factors; previous experiences, the immediate environment, relationships, health and so on.

As Hagrid and Jaffa's confidence grew with one another, we needed to make continual alterations to enable them to flourish. It's a beautiful process to observe. The effort involved in making minor adjustments and the small steps of progress make the world of difference to the big picture. I felt protective toward Jaffa and had not yet bonded with Hagrid, although I liked him and wanted to help him settle. My loyalties were first and foremost with her and I didn't like it if Hagrid walked into her. Naturally she didn't like it either! When a dog is distressed or had health issues, as he did, they can seem disconnected and seemingly have little regard for others, but may not necessarily do it on purpose. As we got to know Hagrid, we learnt about his clumsiness, and that was part of who he was.

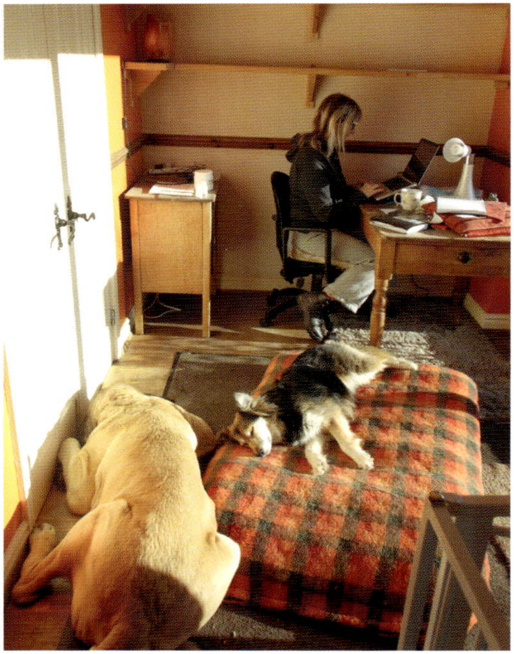

Different dogs and cats learned to relax together while we spent time being around each other.

Communication between animals can be subtle. Hagrid had previously lived with other dogs and learned how to look after himself to an extent. With Jaffa, he was in a new situation, with a smaller dog where he could use his size to get his point across. It was likely that he would use what he'd learned from his past experiences with other dogs and humans. I know that he'd been intimidated, had his attempts at communication ignored, his space invaded and was punished at times. All this can happen when people are unaware of canine language. Sometimes when dogs live together, there can be elements of coercion for survival's sake, and this can be so subtle that we miss it. When a dog has been bullied, showing insecure behaviours that threaten others, they can go on to do what's been done to them. We knew Hagrid had been threatened from at least one other dog in his previous home, and this was one of the reasons he came to live with us.

When he came too close to Jaffa I would casually walk between them, doing it several times until he understood. This is known as splitting up and something dogs do naturally. It gave them a chance to move away from each other and helped them feel more secure. I didn't need to say anything to Hagrid. Each time I felt he might overwhelm Jaffa I'd quietly walk in between them.

Dogs can learn something when we repeat it and are consistent, especially when it's done calmly. Being frustrated or angry would have given him a negative experience and detracted from the relationship we were developing. Besides, he was such a sensitive dog who already had bad experiences, so I wanted to use simple body language to communicate that specific actions weren't acceptable, a language that dogs use and understand.

Being vigilant and consistently repeating the splitting up process before something was about to happen gave Hagrid a chance to learn a different behaviour. Later into their relationship, Hagrid and Jaffa were much more comfortable with each other and could spend more time together.

Being with another dog for a long time can be difficult, so they had times when they were apart during the first few months. This took any pressure off them as they developed the skills to take themselves away when they needed to.

Hagrid had the choice of going into the garden whenever he went near to the door, at first on the lead then later, when he felt safer, on his own. By observing Hagrid's communication and actions, I was able to see when he needed to go outside. The support from the lead and me being there gave him security, which helps dogs enormously in the initial settling-in period.

Lots of dogs are left outside, alone for too long and resort to barking, which as well as becoming a habit is usually a sign they're concerned about something. Some will urinate and defecate indoors after being outside due to being alone and/or too worried to toilet in the garden. For Hagrid, being on lead outside lasted a few weeks as he became used to smells, the neighbours, their routines, dogs and cats in different gardens, regular goings on in the immediate environment such as bin collections, and so on. There was a connection between us via the lead, a nurturing tool to let him know I was there. Being able to run all over the place would have been too much freedom and space, making him overexcited and reactive. However, I noticed that Hagrid was often in conflict while adapting to us. He lacked confidence in many ways and seemed to want to be close, but needed the choice to be able to go away as well. This is one way in which he showed how insecure he was. I used my body language to take the pressure off by standing side-on to him, averting my gaze when he stopped to sniff or faced me. That helped him feel more at ease.

After a few weeks, he was staying inside more and I felt we started to have a connection. When I was around, Hagrid was responsive and reacted to his environment. But when I wasn't, he would lay low and be quiet; something I would imagine he'd learnt as a puppy. Some dogs who have had negative experiences during puppyhood can revert to this kind of shut-down behaviour when they feel worried or uncomfortable. Quite often, this is considered 'good', or at least unobtrusive, behaviour. It's tempting to put a dog like this into situations in which they're uncomfortable, because they appear to give the impression that everything's okay. Sadly it often isn't.

Although it seems counterintuitive, dogs who react by barking, rather than being unreactive and quiet, can have their needs responded to better. If a dog barks, especially a larger one, most people would be scared and give him some space. If a dog doesn't do anything, people are likely to think he is fine and may approach and fuss him. Generally, if they want to be left alone, the dog who barks might get what he wants, and the dog who doesn't bark suffers for it. You can see why they learn to become vocal and reactive. Dogs often just want to communicate, but their silent communication gets missed and/or misunderstood.

Unfortunately there's a chance that a reactive dog could be punished, which obviously isn't a better deal. Conversely, quiet dogs, having their needs ignored, are also under pressure, which can result in them suddenly snapping for 'no reason'. In my experience, this has happened quite a few times; a dog bites for 'no reason' because their communication hasn't been there or hasn't been recognised. Some dogs suffer from health issues as a

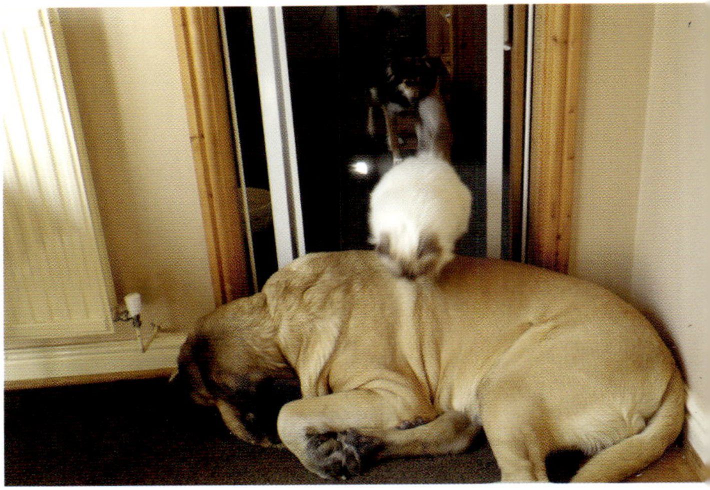

These two had a great relationship. Hagrid was always gentle with Lillibelle the cat and she knew to watch where he walked. She even felt comfortable enough to jump over him! She'd regularly choose to lie and sleep near Hagrid, and they'd gently sniff each other.

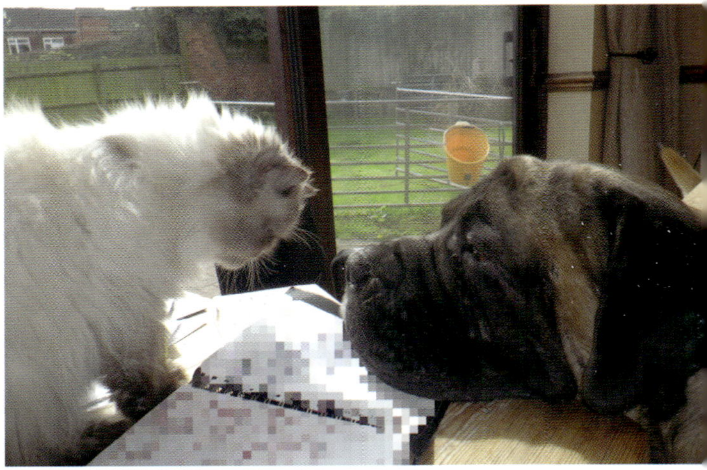

Lillibelle always enjoyed Hagrid's company. He was her kind of dog. They gently sniffed each other as shown here, which was taken on my desk.

result of suppressing emotions and being unreactive, in the same way that humans can.

Hagrid hadn't been familiar with cats, but he became good friends with all of ours. They liked spending time with him, especially Lillibelle. The cats knew when to be around. As mentioned before, at first we used gates so that Hagrid was able to see the cats and his reaction gave them answers as to whether he would be okay with them. They too had choices and were okay with getting close. I've found that most animals get along and find some common ground if boundaries are used, time is given, and they have a balanced lifestyle and choices.

Our relationship

As well as flourishing relationships with the animals in the household, I'm sure Hagrid and I developed a bond because of the shown interest in his needs, by being there for him and listening. Having a towel placed on my lap or shoulder was the first step before interactions began. Each day Hagrid required his eyes wiping (usually several times a day) and the first time was when I came downstairs each day. We'd often sit quietly together in the mornings, both waking up slowly. Hagrid sniffed my eyes while we shared those special minutes together, almost as though he was checking how I was that day.

Most evenings, Hagrid chose to come into the lounge when we settled down and this was another time we shared. He'd rest his head on my lap.

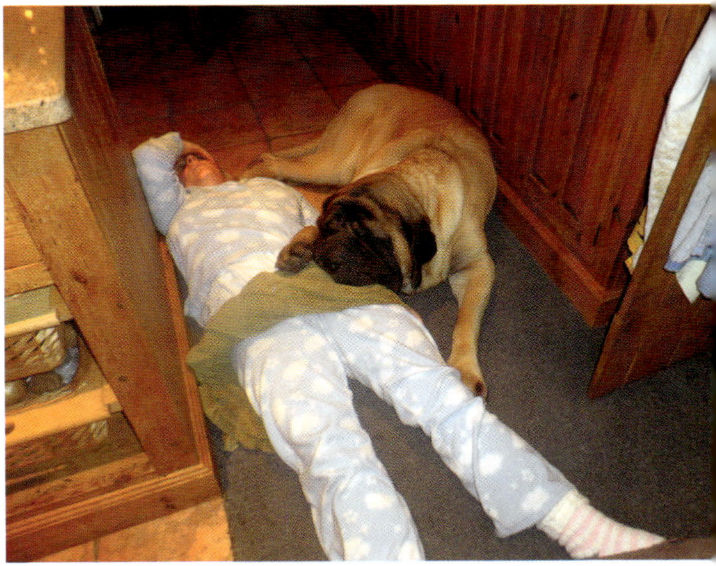

Waking up slowly. Note the towel, these were used for various reasons. I can appreciate that people don't always like slobber on them, hence having a supply of towels and then everyone can relax. A towel placed on our laps ensured Hagrid could do what he naturally needed or wanted to do without us objecting. After all, he wouldn't understand if someone were to recoil every time he approached.

Given a relaxed home environment and a stable foundation with support from their carers, a dog is more likely to be able to deal with the occasional challenging environment. This is true especially if they're exposed to small discomforts at enough of a distance for them to be able to use their communication. When Kaos, a previous Mastiff, was a puppy I thought I needed to train and socialise her, and I was under the impression that this should be done before a certain age. My eagerness and fear, coupled with the short amount of time when socialisation was to happen, only gave a narrow window of opportunity for everything to which she was expected to adjust.

I began to take Kaos to various places so that she would see and meet a variety of people, dogs, animals, traffic and anything else. The result was that she had too much exposure too soon, and too close for her, even though at first she seemed to be okay with some of it. But as she matured, suddenly she started to react to lots of things. In my experience, this can be fairly common. When I sought help to understand her, I learned then that I'd missed a lot of subtle communication. On familiar territory Kaos reacted to people and dogs due to her being worried. In reality, she'd become really scared when I'd been socialising her but wasn't always able to express this because she was overwhelmed and wasn't secure enough in unfamiliar places. I hadn't understood her and had pushed things too close for comfort.

As I mentioned, when Hagrid first came to live with us we limited his world, ensuring he felt safe with the small space he was in. This was quite a different approach to the one I'd used for Kaos. The space he had was two rooms in the house, and on-lead in the garden to begin with. After several weeks he was able to be off-lead in the garden sometimes. We still stayed with him and brought him in after a little while because like most dogs, he needed support while adapting.

Going slowly built his confidence gradually so he wasn't suddenly left to go it alone. A similar process is described in the 'Water' chapter. For Hagrid this was the template with all he came across; people, horses, sheep, traffic and dogs; and how his confidence began to develop.

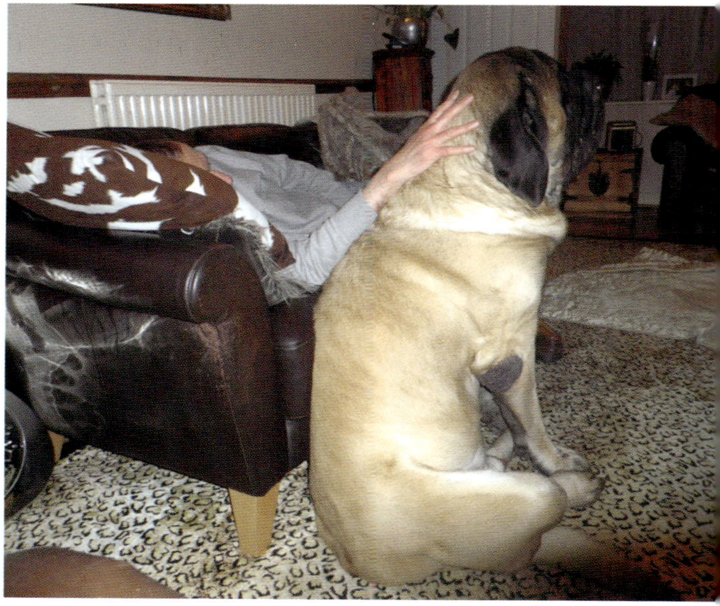

Hagrid would come to Colin for attention only while he was lying down. It seemed that Hagrid could only trust him at a lower level. It needed to be on Hagrid's terms for it to begin.

Dogs in a human world

We didn't need Hagrid to go with us to the town centre, on public transport, to people's parties, and he really didn't need to go either. These were times he could stay at home or in the van and feel more comfortable there. I always ask myself if it's necessary that my dogs need to be involved in these things and who it's for.

Generally, humans tend to have a much faster pace of life than dogs. Because of this, dogs are often rushed around when they need to be given time and space from situations. This can mean going back a few steps and waiting a few days or so for them to regain confidence before going into other scenarios. Dogs vary and will naturally have different levels of assurance. I find it best to take time with them, stay at a distance while observing their language and go at their pace.

For Hagrid, I made sure all exposures to new situations were at a good distance so he could display communication signals and I could have an idea how he felt. Hagrid had been familiar with many other dogs being around him and was used to being with people, so you might think he was properly 'socialised' with them. However, he was considerably worried by both people and dogs. In situations with a lot of dogs, reacting to one of them is a risky thing to do. The whole group could turn on him. When faced with this, dogs may choose to internalise their feelings and the longer that goes on, the more likely it is for them to develop problems.

Is it fair to expect any dog to be immediately at ease in human environments? Maybe for some now and then according to their experience and skills, but regularly enduring human events is probably something we don't want them to have to do if it is negative for them. It's important to observe and note their communication at all times.

Imagine being continually forced or coerced into uncomfortable social situations that you don't want to be in. Having choices and the option to go or not is what would help us, also to take regular breaks, and the same applies for our dogs. In my experience, socialising in this way, with choice, gives dogs much more control over their lives, meaning that they're balanced and that we're creating a relationship based on trust and understanding.

It's worth imagining planning something to put into practice if a difficult scenario arises. Remaining calm is always really helpful, as is giving a dog the distance he needs to be at ease. Dogs respond differently to each dog they see, so they may show interest in a few and not in others. Consider following another dog for a few seconds if it's appropriate, or longer if the dog seems comfortable with a large space between them, so both are at ease.

The degree of exposure will depend on the dog's response. Some like to have information about a few they've seen, and others really would rather not follow the scent of another dog. As with us, they have preferences with those they like. Sometimes walking parallel for a short time, again with plenty of distance between them, helps some dogs deal with others. This used to work for Hagrid when we introduced him to other dogs I knew, who were steady and calm. I'd keep an eye on both as they communicated with one another at a distance.

Dogs meeting can often be our agenda, and not always theirs. There are, of course, dogs who are fine to meet others. How do our dogs, or we, know what the other is like, and what their experiences have been? What might they learn from a meeting?

> By learning to read dogs, we have a much better chance to gauge whether it's suitable for them to meet another.

An example: Kuzu was on a long line at the beach. Another, excitable large dog came bounding over from far away. The approaching dog put its front legs on top of Kuzu, and he retaliated. Next time Kuzu was walked (on-lead) and met another dog, he put his front legs on top of the one he'd just met. That one happened to be a dog he'd interacted with several times previously without needing to do that; before the incident on the beach he'd never done that. Dogs learn from experiences, just as we do. Having positive experiences helps them to take that into other encounters.

Most dogs like to meet others occasionally, especially when they're both relaxed and have had some good experiences to build upon. Given the opportunity, quite a few will choose to avoid others and prefer to observe from a distance. This is when they can take in information and make sensible choices. Those with limited skills may choose to approach a dog and deal with it by bouncing around, for example. Kuzu does that when they worry him, especially when a dog is coming head-on.

The focus is often on our dogs when they meet others. They can sense where our attention is, and in these situations it can be unnaturally intense, which in itself puts pressure on them. When animals are given boundaries, time and don't have these pressures, they can learn what they need to do. They can be slower, relaxed, and get there if they both choose, when we stay more in the background; with them, supportive and casually observing.

It's far better for some to have one or two quality friends they see now and then, rather than a lot of quick interactions that are potentially problematic if they don't have the appropriate skills. They're likely to develop a lack of confidence and/or rush to other dogs, intimidate them, run away, or use other unwanted behaviours. I feel there's often a lot of emphasis on meeting and having to do things with our dogs. Perhaps it's become slightly out of balance. Are we, in effect, trying too hard? I know that was the case for me. By taking a more natural approach with my dogs, over time they've gained the skills to be accepting of other dogs, choosing which ones to meet and those to avoid.

Because I kept a diary for Hagrid, which was always useful in tracking progress, I was able to see that some events had a direct impact on his health, such as visits to the vet, walking too far, hot weather, and when I spent time away from home overnight. With this knowledge I was able to change the way I planned life for him. Some changes were made so that there was more space in between these occasions. This also meant limiting time when I was away, sometimes shortening walks, either staying inside during hot weather or choosing cooler times of the day to go out. I would be careful not to go to the vet unnecessarily, and planned how it was done. And the vet was happy to talk about problems on the phone, assessing whether it was necessary to take Hagrid into the surgery.

By doing these things for him in order to avoid negative situations, our trust was strengthened.

Key points

- It can take dogs approximately up to a year to fully settle in, depending on previous experiences, health and so on. For that reason, it was necessary to give both our dogs space of their own, be mindful of their communication, and the development of their relationship.
- As their confidence grew with one another, we made continual alterations to enable them to flourish.
- When Hagrid came too close to Jaffa I would casually walk between them, doing it several times until he understood. This is known as splitting up and something dogs do naturally.
- Being vigilant and consistently repeating the splitting up process before something was about to happen gave Hagrid chances to learn a different behaviour.

Key points (continued)

- Living and being with another dog for a long time can be difficult, so early on they had times when they were apart. This takes pressure off them as they develop skills to take themselves away.
- Quiet dogs can snap for 'no reason' if their needs are ignored, or feel under pressure.
- I used my body language to take pressure off Hagrid and make him more at ease by standing side-on, and averting my gaze when he stopped to sniff, or faced me.
- Support from the lead delivers security, which helps dogs enormously in the initial settling-in period.
- Some dogs suffer from health issues as a result of suppressing emotions and being unreactive; similar to humans.
- Kaos had become scared when I'd been socialising her but wasn't always able to express this because she didn't feel secure enough in unfamiliar places.
- Given a relaxed home environment, a stable foundation with support from their carers, a dog is more likely to be able to deal with the occasional challenging environment.
- I always consider if it's necessary that dogs need to be involved in my social situations.
- In my experience, giving appropriate choice offers dogs much more control over their lives, meaning that they're balanced and that we're creating a relationship based on trust and understanding.
- Dogs learn from experiences, just as we do. Having positive experiences helps a dog to take that into other encounters.
- Keeping a diary for Hagrid was always useful in tracking progress. I was able to see that some events had a direct impact on his health, such as visits to the vet, walking too far, hot weather, and when I spent time away from home.

CHAPTER 5

Hagrid's relationship with my grandchildren

I'm including our grandchildren here because they were a large part of Hagrid's life. They visited regularly, sometimes staying a few hours, other times a few days and set the precedent for Hagrid to be able to deal with other visitors who came with children, and of course seeing children out on walks. Youngsters can be great for dogs, provided boundaries and barriers, appropriate for the skills of both, are in place.

The most significant reason, however, to include our grandchildren here is that so often it's a dog that's familiar to a child that bites. Therefore, having a few boundaries and barriers and addressing the dog's needs ensures the safety of any children. We're preventing distress for the dog by taking this action.What can happen is the dog's needs are unintentionally put on hold while children visit.

There have been a couple of incidents for us as a family over the years where there's been conflict or near misses with our children and dogs. I'm writing this in the hope that it highlights ways of making life safer and easier for dogs when children are around, whether they're residents or visitors. It's mainly lack of awareness at catering to a dog's needs and an understanding of their language that cause things to go wrong when a child is bitten.

Years ago, my daughter was bitten by my parents' dog. Shandy was a very nervous dog and it was New Year's Eve, which is a time of year lots of dogs are with friends and family for longer periods than usual. Routine is often very different at that time of year and it is for the dogs as well. There are added pressures on them.

Mum and I had been to the sales and just come home with bags to be unpacked. The kettle was on as we stood near the doorway from the kitchen to the dining room. I was standing right next to my eleven-month-old daughter, and Shandy by the doorway. My daughter crawled through the kitchen into the dining room when Shandy, who was also walking though the same doorway the other way, jumped on her. I was quick and pulled Shandy off by his collar but in that split second my daughter had needed six stitches in her ear. Shandy was put to sleep as a result of the incident, which has been one of my life's biggest regrets. He was a lovely, sensitive dog who was simply misunderstood and paid the ultimate price.

At that time, over thirty-five years ago, dogs were routinely put to sleep for biting people; they were supposed to get on with people, full stop. To my horror, dogs today are still put to sleep for the same reasons. It seems society hasn't changed much in all those years. That is such a shame.

Accidents do happen where the dogs' and children's skills may have been misjudged or not considered, as in the case with Shandy and my daughter. At the time, my Mum and I were chatting, with half an eye on the toddler and Shandy. The way we as a family do things now is different and both have clear boundaries, which keeps them safe.

Statistics show that children are often bitten by a known dog. I know of several cases where a visiting child has been bitten by the family dog. But we all know how it can be when there's a lot going on. It's easy to lose focus when humans and dogs are all together during a visit and the children are left with the dog while the adults chat. This puts a lot of pressure on the dog, especially without regular breaks, appropriate supervision and consideration.

Perhaps in some cases, dogs are seen as being a minor consideration, of less importance. I'd like to challenge that belief and bring their needs into the foreground. There's bound to be a problem if on the one hand they receive attention most days, then suddenly visitors and children are there and the dog receives inappropriate attention or none when it's needed. Moreover, they may be restricted and even reprimanded for what might be usual dog behaviour, or if they growl. There are most likely to have been other signals before this. A growl is a dog's way of saying they've had enough, are worried, and need more space. Dogs are often expected to behave impeccably; and interestingly, more so than a child!

Sometimes it seems as though children, because we understand them more, have freedom and dogs have far less than usual. There are likely to be problems if this happens, and it is my aim to raise awareness of a few small changes that can minimise disruption and risk.

There was an incident with Hagrid while I was out one day. People were chatting in the kitchen, with Hagrid and William, our grandson, there. Suddenly Hagrid air-snapped, just missing William. Even though the people there were aware of the boundaries I needed for Hagrid and the children, they thought they were unnecessary because Hagrid appeared to be a well-behaved dog. It wasn't clear that he was in a state where that might happen.

Everyone learns in their own way, but it can be at a high cost to the dog. We took some precautionary steps with Hagrid and the children. Ahead of the visit, the children were made aware of the boundaries. On the day, dogs and children were given regular breaks, which meant time apart so they had relief from one another and a change of environment.

With care and thought, we established a harmonious balance between both the children's and the dogs' needs. In fact, these complemented one another, and a strong, positive relationship was formed. Children learn to understand and consider the needs and feelings of another being when it is explained to them, which is a wonderful opportunity for them on their journey toward adulthood.

As grandparents, we helped in the organisation of a routine that worked for everyone. As a family, we varied what we did. Sometimes we'd be in the house doing things together, and at other times the children were able to wait a short while for their turn for attention, which was another learning opportunity.

Our dogs are our responsibility every day, and if I suddenly put others' needs before theirs, they could quickly become jealous, anxious, or reactive, which has potential to put the children in jeopardy.

When family visits, I keep the dogs' routines as stable as possible while still being flexible, which means the dogs are fulfilled. The time and focus leave me available to devote time to our family and grandchildren and most importantly this keeps them safe. I love them deeply and because they feel safe and secure, they are in a position to learn about the dogs.

Our grandchildren have grown up with our dogs but haven't always had access to them. That's been a gradual process. We always take on rescue dogs (Kaos was the one exception) and have barriers in place while they adjust to one another over time. Each day, I take into account both the children and the dog's mood and state of health, then decide when or if it's okay for them to spend time together.

Planning ahead means there are opportunities to slowly change the routine so that the dogs are prepared for the children's visit. For example if walks are going to be at a different time of day, this can be incorporated into their routine ahead of the event. I realise that not everyone is in a position to make these changes but some small ones can often be made, depending on the individual circumstances.

We talked with the children about the reasons why our dogs' needs are important. They've gradually been involved in their health and welfare, and enjoy joining in and helping with walking and feeding them, as far as their skills allow. That's why it works so well.

Being over-excited without rules or boundaries doesn't work so well, and we tended to avoid overly stimulating activities when the dogs were around. I remember one time we played a loud, fun game called 'Snorta', a memory game played by making animal noises. The dogs were resting in another room and I kept an eye on them regularly. It was pleasantly surprising how well they dealt with it. We only played this game when the dogs were already used to the children's visits and wouldn't have played it if the dogs were affected by the excitement. Part of this is that our dogs' stress levels are monitored, so we're aware of what causes them distress, and limit this as much as possible. If something does happen, their tolerance is higher than it would be if they were constantly aroused by exciting games, exercise and disruption. It's like people really: if we're constantly bombarded with stimulus or have a lot of stress in our lives, our ability to deal with simple situations becomes more strained and our judgement can become impaired.

When the children were younger, between three and six years old, lots of the time was spent in the bath, not necessarily around bedtime. Those with children or grandchildren of their own will know that quite a few of them love playing in water. Many happy hours were spent in the bathroom and the dogs were happy downstairs having time off. It can be tiring for dogs, not just adults, to have young children around for any length of time, so that time off really helped our dogs.

Children may require a lot of attention, and there are ways to deal with this that keeps everyone happy. When the children were young we'd often meet up somewhere with family, leaving the dogs at home, which was an opportunity for them to rest. When we came back they were calm and relaxed. Sometimes, we'd bring the children back home with us.

Other times we'd meet at our house for a while and then go out, leaving the dogs at home to sleep for a few hours. They needed time to rest after family or visitors had come around. When we met at our house, at first the dogs would be in another room, one of us with them. This is because arrivals and departures are generally exciting times, so giving our dogs space can be necessary until they've adapted to the new situation. Keeping them separate from the 'action' lets the excitement pass, and once everything has calmed down and the children are happily playing quietly, it may be good for the dog to come in if he wants to.

At times we'd also bring the dogs in individually on a long line, provided they were used to being on the lead without that in itself getting them more excited. Just a few seconds in the room at first would be enough, then they'd be happy to be taken out again. How long they were in the room would depend on their communication and ability to deal with the situation. Some dogs will be fine to come into a room without a lead as some of ours have been, but using a lead is how we did it with those who would benefit from the security at the outset.

Having regular breaks was very important for our dogs to give them a breather. For us, this included being with them outside while they pottered around calmly, had a break and a chance to sniff around and de-stress.

Hagrid's first experiences with my grandchildren

Colin and I took steps to settle Hagrid into our family. At first, we met up with them at local garden centres or at other people's houses while Hagrid was becoming familiar with us. For many dogs, meeting lots of people in the first few days/weeks can be overwhelming, so we took it easy. As mentioned, my grandchildren often visited so I wanted to get this right and make sure they and Hagrid felt settled before they were introduced for short times. Katey, my granddaughter, was a little concerned by Hagrid's size at first. She was two and a half years old and roughly the same height as Hagrid at that point. You can imagine that could be daunting.

When they came to visit, family would sit and chat in the lounge at first, away from Hagrid but he could still see them through a dog gate. One of us would stay with him for some of the time, especially when he was getting to know everyone.

It can be a good idea to meet a new person while out on a walk, which is occasionally what we did with Hagrid, and it worked well. That meant he had outside distractions that he could use by sniffing and exploring, and didn't need to deal with the person. He could put his attention on something else, which helped him deal with the situation.

During the walk, Hagrid would gain confidence to sniff the person, which was an important part of getting to know them. It can be useful for some dogs to meet someone in this way, and then to enter the house together. Once inside, it may be appropriate for them to be separate rather than allow pressure to build, depending on the dog and the particular visitor. Later, it may be possible for them to be in the same room together. This approach provides for a more relaxed meeting, rather than having new people suddenly arrive at the door, with all the excitement and anxiety that can bring. Every dog is different, as are people, so the interactions between them will vary.

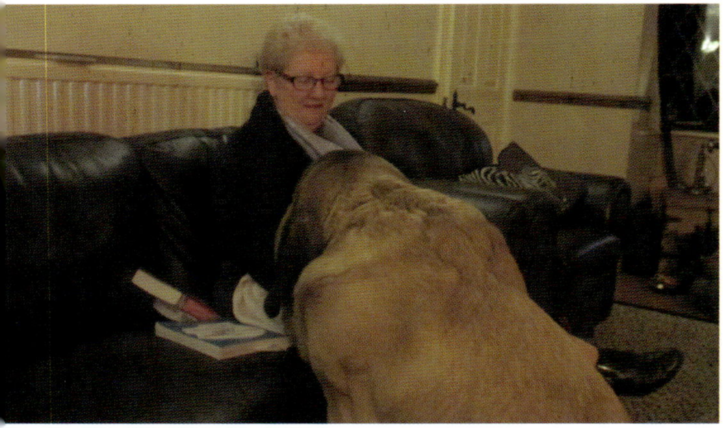

Our visitor, Sue, is a good friend I could trust to take a hands-off approach. When she arrived, we settled down and had a drink and a chat, with Hagrid and I sitting behind a gate, meaning he could observe and gather information about her. Then, once we were all relaxed, Hagrid was able to saunter into the room and inspect her, then he just went to lie down.

For quite a few dogs, being introduced to someone who's sitting down can be more comfortable especially if they can carry on talking to other people in the room and leave the dog alone. This made it much easier for Hagrid to walk away when he chose to, because the focus was not on him.

If introduced while sitting down, and because Hagrid was unsure of people, we found it best to take him out before the visitor stood up. Some dogs can become worried when strangers get up unexpectedly and start moving around.

We used the same approach for the children, so they were frequently sitting at the table involved in an activity. Having something quiet and calm to occupy them proved to be a good idea. Also, an adult being engaged with the children would take the focus off the dog for those first moments, and reduced excitement. The aim is for the dog to come in, and have the act not be a big deal. The less fuss made of it, the better.

Playhouses were often out for the children. Books and other quiet toys helped to encourage a calm atmosphere. Usually, an adult was available to interact with them as they played, which helps children to feel included and cared for. I often tried to spend my time with the dogs initially, until they were settled, then with the children, but I realise this isn't always possible for everyone to do.

Another factor that is worth mentioning is that the children were used to dogs, so rather than being drawn to them as a novelty, they accepted the animal being there as part of everyday life. That helped as it had a very natural feel.

Katey

In the first few months, when Hagrid was still in the throes of settling in, my granddaughter Katey would sit on the kitchen table if my daughter came in to chat with me. That way, she and Hagrid slowly adapted to being around each other. She was safe and felt secure by being on the table, and Hagrid got used to her just by them being around together like that. Katey gained confidence as she watched Hagrid, and he gained confidence from knowing her. Any low-key, relatively quiet activity like this helped to build up both the children's and dog's confidence.

My granddaughter is generally calm and quiet. She's easy-going and her attitude to life and ability to observe is met with respect from animals. She didn't attempt to reach out to stroke Hagrid, and many animals prefer people to leave them alone. That's especially true with someone they don't know well, which encourages a shared relationship. Because she was small, Katey usually stood on chairs while helping me cook and wash up in the kitchen.

Boundaries such as closed gates were in place, so Hagrid was in a different room but able to see from where he was. The gates were there to give the children and Hagrid space of their own, and it's also something a dog can understand clearly as opposed to me telling him what to do.

Sometimes Hagrid joined us, depending on what was going on. Mostly he came in with the two of us for short stints, and could see what we were doing before I took him into his room or the hallway to watch from there. Hagrid went into another room because it's not always possible to concentrate fully on cooking with a child and keeping an eye on them both.

To be able to use gates effectively, our dogs needed to be familiar with them first, so using them ahead of when they were required - for very short periods - added to their success and reduced frustration for the dogs. They became used to these boundaries, though as time went by, Hagrid and the children learned not to need them because they were at ease with each other.

When Katey was old enough, she was asking to join me on walks with the dogs. I was able to teach her a lot. Hagrid was slow, making it easy for Katey to keep up, and he didn't walk too far either so again, they were well suited. Their inner speed complemented each other's.

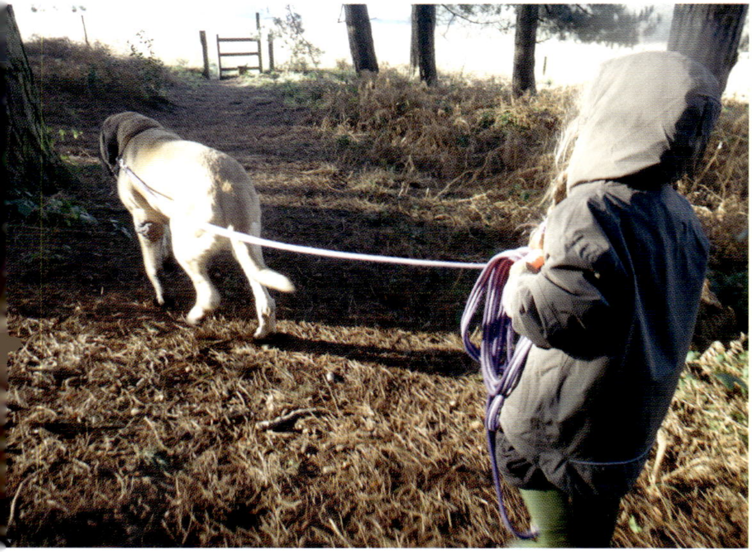

Katey and Hagrid on a walk. When not much was going on, it was possible to teach Katey (who was seven at the time) a few simple ways of handling (walking) a dog. Hagrid was happy to have Katey walk slowly behind him and she learnt how it felt to draw the lead in and out when needed. She got a feel for walking Hagrid. The experience lasted maybe a couple of minutes but I was there, able to guide and give support to both of them when they needed, without putting pressure on either one.

Resting at a stile before heading back through the woods. For a few minutes we had a break, enjoying the day. Hagrid chose to sit next to Katey. It's interesting to note that he sat side on to her, and she held her head and face away from him, avoiding direct eye contact. Positioning counts for a lot with animals and recognising its importance is fascinating. At one point Hagrid sniffed Katey's face, something dogs we know well like to do. She just let him. The two of them were at ease with one another, which I took into account before taking the photo.

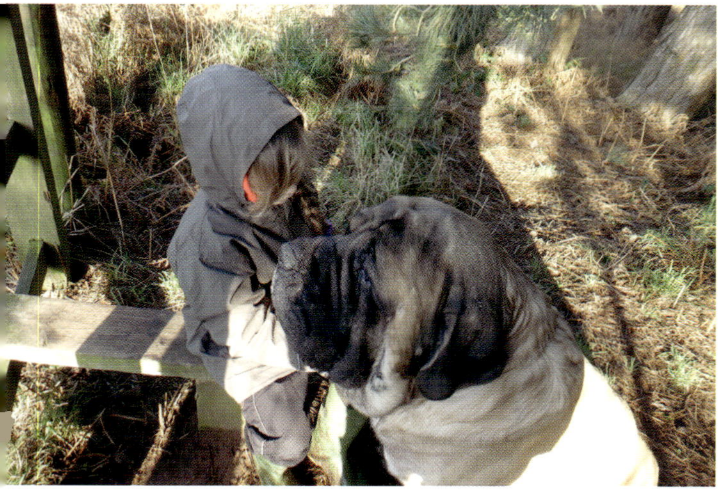

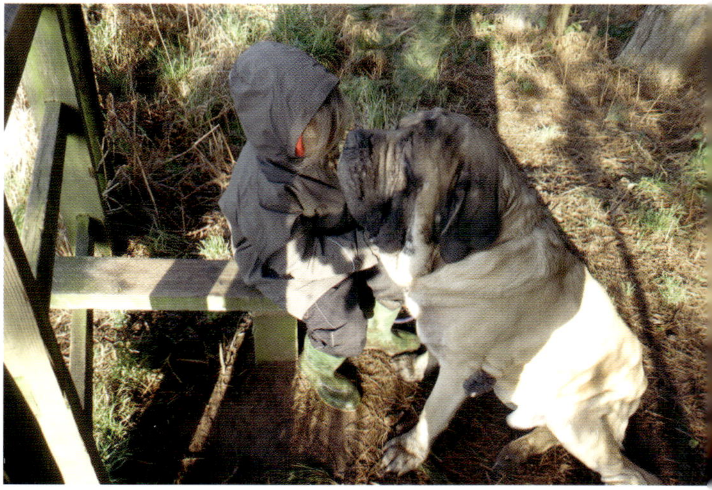

William

While William, my grandson, showed interest in dogs at times, he wasn't always as keen as Katey. This in itself was positive, because he would leave the dogs alone and get on with other things.

As William matured he became more interested in the dogs and came with me on some walks, often asking questions about aspects of my life with them and, surprisingly, a significant amount of the way we live with our pets influenced him with his own dog. He applied what he learnt, and saw how it helped Comet, their Cavalier. Although William hasn't always shown an interest in dogs, he learnt enough to put appropriate changes in place for Comet, and even passed on some of this knowledge to his parents. By our actions, we can influence others even if we're not always aware of it.

Now and then William asked to come with us on Sunday mornings, as the children often like to come when I take a dog out. We also have walks with them, without the dogs. Then it's the children's walk.

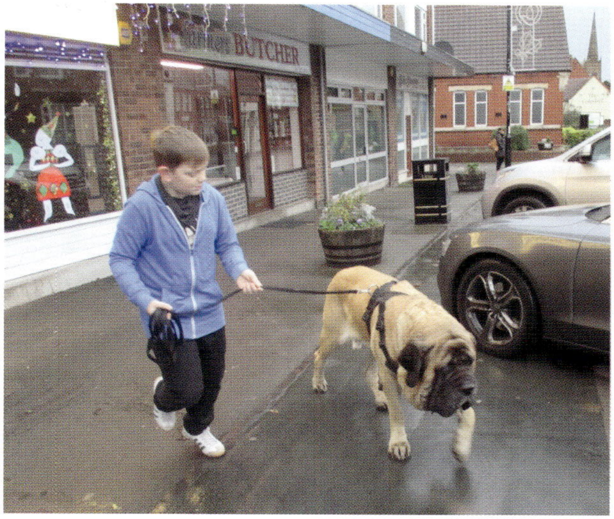

A quiet Sunday morning walk with William, Hagrid and myself when there was hardly any traffic around. For short times William was able to handle Hagrid with my guidance. Note how William watches Hagrid so he can gauge what to do next. 'Being' with a dog on a walk is really important for building bonds and working together. Children can be very responsible if allowed short times to practice caring for another and learning new skills. They enjoy it and it teaches them respect for animals.

Before leaving the house, I explained to William that this was Hagrid's walk and he would need to walk with me, behind him because many dogs worry about children being ahead of them. William wanted to bring a football with him, but I said that we'd play football later. Kicking a football around on a walk with most dogs is likely to overexcite and worry them, which can lead to undesirable behaviours.

On a different occasion, we were taking Pogo out for a walk and William wanted to come on his scooter. This was fine for her, as he was mindful to stay behind. The walk worked well and Pogo settled comfortably, enjoying her time with William safely behind. Some dogs and children would be okay with this, and others might not. In this case, both had the ability to deal with it.

Now William's older, he has the skills to be able to show some restraint whilst still being able to enjoy walks with us. By being clear on the boundaries, he has the choice whether he wants to come or not. My grandchildren enjoy the walks we have with the dogs and choose when they join us. And of course, it's an opportunity for them to learn respect for other living beings and to have empathy for their needs and feelings.

Likewise, Katey enjoys helping me with Zoopharmacognosy sessions (see the chapter on Health) and learnt about canine communication, understanding the tiny movements dogs make such as blinking, changes in breathing patterns, ear twitches and so on. With Hagrid, we did this together, and she had time to understand him. Katey also helped prepare the dog's vegetables as we put them in the juicer, mixing juice and pulp together with her bare hands. I always saved that for her when she visited.

Zoopharmacognosy enables captive or domesticated animals to use self-medicative behaviour by offering plant extracts that contain the same, or similar components to those found in an animal's natural environment. There's more explanation in the chapter on Health.

Because of how we approached everything between the children and the dogs, the relationship was safe for both of them, so they were able to build a bond based on trust and respect. The children have always respected the dogs' need for space and only interacted with them if the dogs showed they wanted to. It was important the children didn't wander up to and interact with the dogs because they felt like it. I've seen other children doing this, even when a dog is worried or sleeping.

Children don't always know what's acceptable to animals unless adults guide them from the start. They can be taught to understand some simple rules, and be supported as they learn. It's important to keep them safe.

Key points

- Youngsters can be great for dogs, provided boundaries and barriers, appropriate for the skills of both, are in place.
- Addressing the dog's needs ensures the safety of children and prevents distress for the dog.
- It's easy to lose focus when humans and dogs are all together during a visit and the children are left with the dog. This puts a lot of pressure on a dog.
- Our grandchildren have grown up with our dogs but haven't always had access to them. That's been a gradual process.
- Having regular breaks was very important for our dogs to give them a breather. This included being with them outside while they pottered around calmly. These short activities gave them a break, a chance to sniff around and de-stress.
- Katey didn't attempt to reach out to stroke Hagrid, and many animals prefer people to leave them alone. That's especially true with someone they don't know well.
- Gates keep children safe and give dogs their own space: they're also something a dog can understand clearly instead of being told what to do.
- My grandchildren enjoy the walks we have with the dogs and choose when they join us. It's an opportunity for them to learn respect for other living beings and to have empathy for their needs and feelings.
- It was important the children didn't wander up to and interact with the dogs because they felt like it.
- Children don't always know what's acceptable to animals unless adults guide them from the start. They can be taught to understand some simple rules and be supported as they learn.

Chapter 6

Health and appearance

When I talk about using appearance to determine the health of a dog, I'm using the term in its widest sense. There is so much that can be gained from taking a holistic approach and using all senses to assess a dog's health. It's worth beginning by considering how we know if someone is ill, either physically or mentally, as this can give much insight to transfer over to understanding dogs.

Instinctively it's possible to tell if someone is ill, by observing them or by using our other senses such as hearing, touch and smell. Intuition can tell us something is different, even though it may not always be evident what at the time. As humans, we're accustomed to observing people and so generally have a good sense of what is 'normal' for someone regarding their health.

Signs that someone is unwell are:

- They stay in bed all day
- Their eyes seem tired
- Their skin looks worn or has a rash
- Their hair may seem different, dull, broken or has dandruff
- They cold be hunched rather than upright
- Their voice sounds different or they find it hard to speak

- They lose interest in day-to-day activities
- They smell different
- They develop lumps, bumps, or sores
- They eat too much or have no appetite at all
- They have an upset stomach
- They tell us!

The same innate intelligence can be used with dogs and the same logic can be applied to animals. However, I've found developing skills in this area takes practice and observation.

For example, there are sheep near us and when I walk in the fields, the lone sheep that are far away from the others, those that are unmoving until the last minute, hunched, holding themselves awkwardly or have dishevelled wool almost always have something wrong with them. Usually it's a combination of these signs that acts as an indicator.

Dogs speak to all of us and let us know when something isn't suiting them, in their own language; it's a matter of learning and understanding the individual.

When a new animal comes into my home, particularly one that I haven't known since they were born, it can take a little longer to get to know them. It is important to spend time being around them to gain a sense of what constitutes normal for any animal. This will differ widely from one to another, so if there's more than one dog, as well as noting them individually, observing both is great as it shows how they behave individually and together. I notice dogs wherever I go, in various settings and trust my senses, remaining open and inquisitive. For example, many people recognise a dog wagging its body from side to side in a relaxed way can be a sign of happiness. What some people don't know is that dogs can also wag their tails before biting, and that a wagging tail doesn't necessarily mean that a dog is friendly or happy.

What really helped me to get a grip on this kind of language was recording in a notebook what I saw. This can become a reference point to which you return. For me, because Hagrid had problems with his skin, I noted what food he was eating, some environmental factors and day-to-day events. After a while, I was able to see some patterns emerge. The more I recorded, the more I saw. This didn't give a definitive answer, but helped in the big scheme of things.

Interestingly, there have been changes in my life that have obviously influenced my dogs' lives. I noted down times when they were enjoying life, as well as when they were finding things more difficult. When one was ill, looking back at the notes was extremely useful for tracing the events leading up to it, which meant with awareness I could avoid the same thing happening in future.

It's worth knowing that both excitement and distress trigger the same chemical reactions in the body. Regularly racing around for more than a few seconds can be a possible contributing factor to injury and illness.

There are inevitably various other reasons why a dog would be racing around other than for enjoyment. Over-excitement can be a stress response to other things happening, and the dog needs to race around to deal with the way he's feeling.

Body language is equally as important when a dog is sleeping as when he is active. How does he usually lie when asleep? This is good to know as changes in sleeping positions may indicate difficulty finding a comfortable position and indicate an underlying health issue early on. Changing sleeping positions was an early sign of Jaffa's heart problem. She began to sleep with her head propped up on something, such as a pillow: it helped her to breathe more easily, opening the airways.

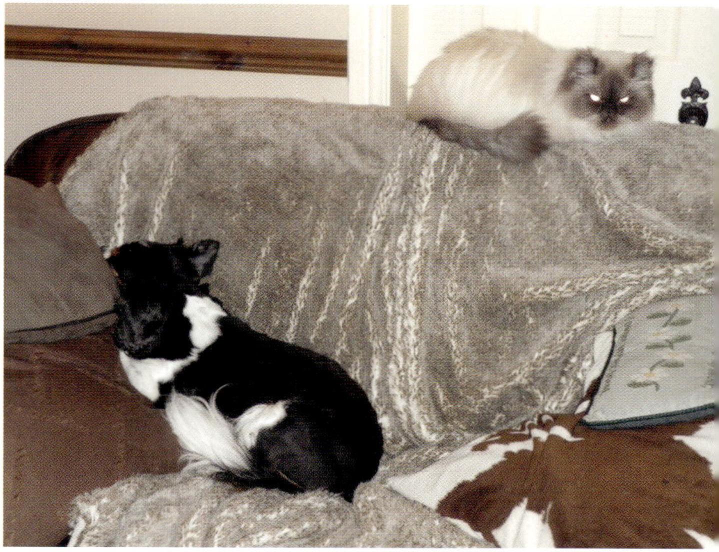

Jaffa began to prop her head up, making it easier for her to breathe. These little changes were indicators for us to find out more and to be able to help her have a more comfortable life. We made sure she had sleeping places where it was possible for her head to be raised and, conscious of her exercise levels, decided shorter walks would be more beneficial. During hot weather we provided her with cool places in the house to rest, and gave her walks very early in the morning, preferably near water.

I'm also reminded of something that worried us about Hagrid's appearance. To start with, I thought he had problems in his back: he had such a noticeable arch that looked considerably rounded. Humans can carry stress and anxiety in their shoulders, with some people appearing to be quite hunched, whereas dogs often carry stress in their legs and lower back.

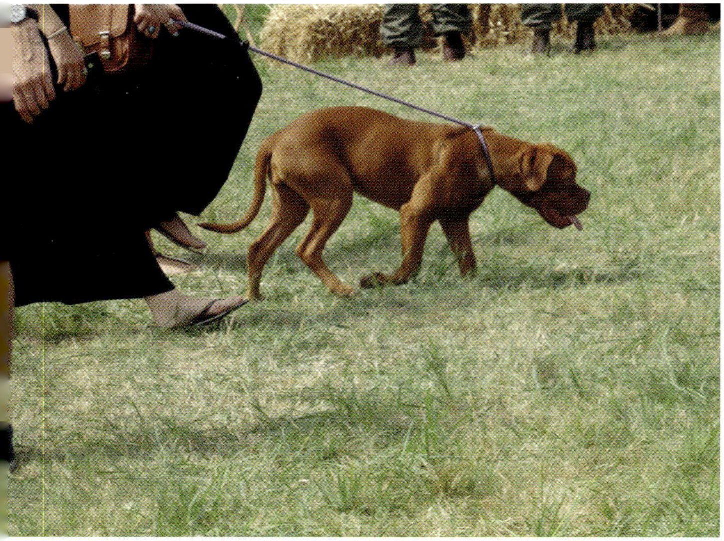

This shows how some dogs carry tension in a tucked under, or 'roached', back end. The photo was taken at a summer fete on a boiling hot day with little shade and was such a struggle for many animals there. The short, restrictive lead shows how limited the dog's choices were, while the dog pulled to try and gain personal space.

Quite a few dogs have some degree of being 'tucked under' and this is something to bear in mind. I hoped that in time, Hagrid's rounded back appearance would flatten out as he became more relaxed. Thankfully, this proved to be the case. In time (a lot of time!) as he was listened to, given choices and respected, he was able to feel settled and, above all, loved. This took about a year in total, with his back changing in shape and becoming much flatter. Eventually Hagrid completely lost the hunched appearance, which was fantastic. He also grew in confidence, and his back legs became stronger in spite of limited exercise.

There are other ways that a dog's appearance shows that they're struggling. Changes or differences might be in their coat that, for example, may change from one particular colour such as brown to various shades of brown. The feel and texture may be different, becoming coarse, patchy, dusty or powdery. A dog's colour or the way their hair lies could be different. There may be a sheen or lack of it; their eyes can be red when they're pushed to the limit and tired, or they can be bright, or dull, as though nothing is behind them. I note any changes in my animals.

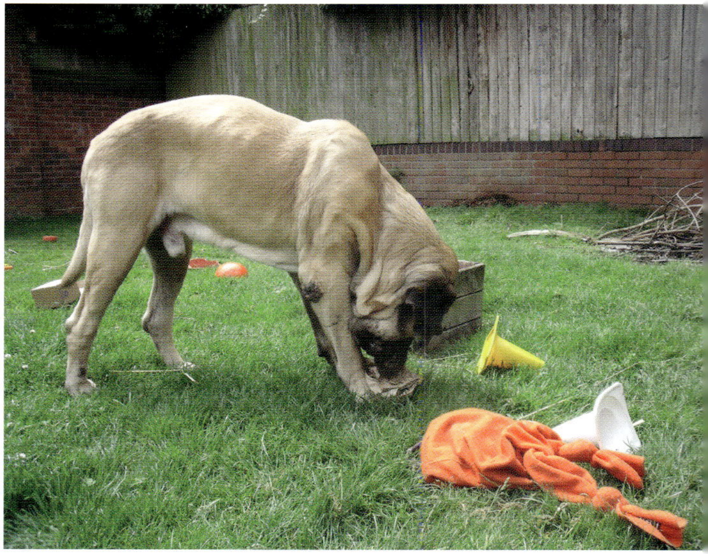

This photo shows Hagrid's roached back. For a good few months this was his shape.

Holding tension

People are very much affected by experiences and the treatment received from others, and this is often reflected in their appearance. For example, someone may hold their head down, turn away, slump their shoulders, make very little eye contact, or avoid it entirely.

Experiences can also affect where and how people position themselves when with others. Some might stay in the background to avoid being noticed because of feeling awkward. There are those who put themselves forward, seemingly extrovert, but may be doing so to compensate for a lack of confidence. The same happens for dogs, and their appearance can be greatly influenced by the way they are treated.

As well as appearance, a dog's behaviour can tell us about their emotional state, how they're feeling and how they've been treated in the past. Seeing the changes in Hagrid's appearance over time as he was nurtured, loved and guided through difficulties was wonderful.

Dogs can be tense in all parts of their bodies, their skin, jaw, mouth, legs, back, tail and paws. The more dogs observed, the better; walking down the street, in the park, at the vet and at home. Is their speed fast, slow, or erratic? Do different surfaces affect them in any way? What is their gait like? Do their legs move in unison? How do they relate to their handler? If something happens, what is the reaction?

There are so many ways a dog can hold tension. First, it's an advantage to know what a dog looks like when totally relaxed, there are visible signs when a dog is tense:

- How does his skin move and lie?
- Is the dog moving with ease or difficulty?
- Do the dog's legs hold their weight evenly?
- How does their tail hang?
- Is the dog's coat neat or rough?
- Is their breathing regular or laboured?
- What are the ears like and how do they hang?
- How does the dog hold his head?
- Are their eyes bright and responsive, or dull and distant?

When we attended a dog show, Kaos, my first Mastiff, would have stiff legs to the point of being completely straight. Her stomach would be tucked under, and her body looked tense. Her back was arched. Looking at photos really shows this.

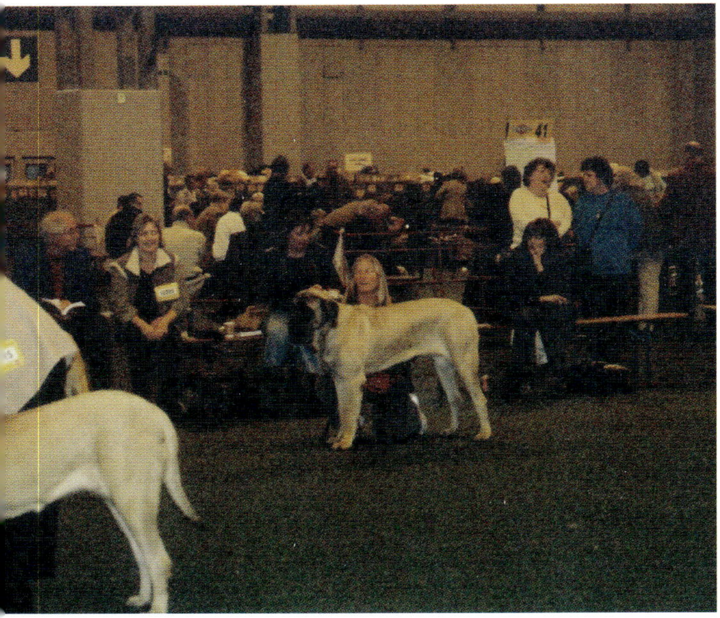

Kaos and I at Crufts, in the centre of the picture. She appears to have a tucked under appearance and her legs are stiff, almost straight, showing the tautness she's holding.

Many dogs struggle at these kinds of events and show it in a variety of ways. Examples could be not reacting, usually referred to as shut down, showing little or no emotion; being highly excited (nervous excitement), making poor decisions and mistakes. Physical signs can be stiffness, drooling, dandruff, moulting, red eyes, panting, diarrhoea, urinating more, not going to the toilet, not eating or drinking, and so on.

Poor Kaos had a terrible day and it was the first time she chased a dog. There was so much going on, too much for her to deal with from an overwhelming number of people and dogs. The outburst with the dog happened towards the end of the day and was completely uncharacteristic for her.

With knowledge, when I consider the events of the day, it's no surprise that she reacted as she did. Sometimes people say behaviours like this, especially biting, are out of character, often because the build-up to this point has gone unnoticed and unrecognised. For a dog in this situation there's enormous pressure and our expectations far exceed what is natural for them. I never took Kaos to another dog show after this because I recognised how traumatic it had been for her.

The way a dog stands can be a good indicator of physical and mental health. How does he carry his weight? Is it evenly balanced over four legs? Are the nails the same length on all four feet or are they worn down unevenly? Are the muscles evenly distributed? Listen to the sound of the dog's feet on the ground. Does he pick all of his feet up when he walks or does one foot scrape on the ground, for example?

Pain can have an impact on appearance and behaviour too. Dogs can pant when they're in pain, however they pant for various reasons. Other factors will be present if there's pain. The way they move might be slower and more deliberate, perhaps taking more care than usual if they're holding tension, or maybe they're conserving energy because of the pain.

Digestive issues and allergies could also be impacting this kind of behaviour. Wind is something Hagrid had during the early days with us and at that time his food didn't suit him. Unsuitable food causes pressure on the body and mind. Dogs can also have wind if they're under pressure, as an exhibitor of stress. Behaviour changes may also be evident.

Of course, a dog's smell isn't strictly appearance, but it can be another clue to what may be going on with their health. I've come to know what my dogs smell like and when there are changes. Hagrid smelt terrible when he first came to live with us. Fortunately, this smell changed for the better as his health improved, and then deteriorated when his inflammation became worse.

Dogs smell different when their coats are wet and at other times in their lives. Their skin, ears, feet and breath can smell, but all of these can change in time and that's why it's an advantage to have a mental and physical note of how a dog is when he's healthy; it provides a baseline.

Dogs' poo can tell us a great deal about them too. For instance, a normal poo is easy to pick up and hardly leaves a trace on the ground. Too hard or too soft possibly means something may not be suiting them, or they're worried in some way, as this can impact on digestion. The number of times a dog poos during a day is also relevant. How many is normal for a particular dog? Does this change in certain situations?

For example, some walks may be different to others. What are the differences in the walks in relation to how much they're pooing or its consistency? How long are the walks? Who is present? What does the dog come across? I consider the environment as well as the dog's body language and communication. What's been going on in previous days? Often, these considerations can point to an accumulation that proves to be too much for the dog. There are several other situations that can influence a dog's digestion in similar ways. Incidentally, on the day Kaos was at Crufts from early in the morning until late afternoon, she didn't poo at all.

Some other signs that may go with poor digestion could be a gurgling stomach, flatulence or the dog being fussy with food when usually he wouldn't be. Perhaps he's reluctant to go for a walk, is more subdued than usual, or his sleeping patterns are different. Alongside all of this, taking the dog's behaviour into consideration is relative. A well-behaved dog who is always good may well be internalising emotions. Has his behaviour changed in any way? Is he grumpy sometimes and/or unpredictable? Communication, body language and health are all connected.

If a dog is erratic, jumping up, chewing on their lead, digging, barking, or displaying irrational behaviour, then he needs to be listened to and taken much further away from the situation, whatever it is. As a rule, I always question what a dog does, and look at the whole picture.

Illness

Please note: within this section there are a few graphic photos of Hagrid's skin, that some may find unpleasant or off-putting.

Hagrid was a dog who was ill for much of his life.

It was just eight days after Hagrid joined our household that we made our first trip to the vets, and at this point we learned so much more about him. We were amazed to see that, at just two and a half years old, he already had five pages of vet notes! This gives an indication to the extent of his health issues.

He'd had two previous operations on his front right leg, and had suffered with eye, skin and ear problems throughout his young life. I was staggered to learn this and so was the vet.

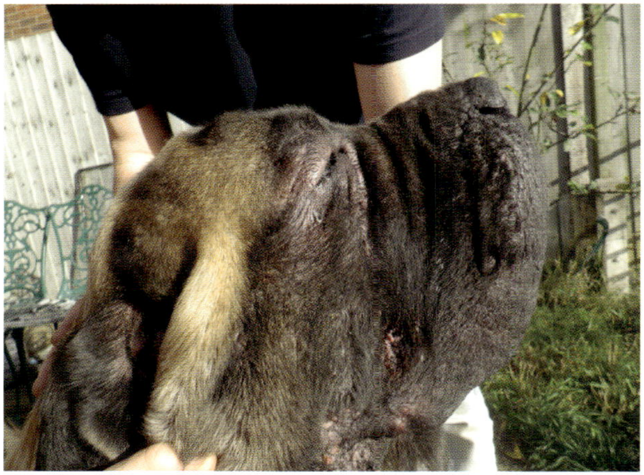

Occasionally, when his skin was continually oozing, I shaved Hagrid's neck and chest – which he was happy to let me do as it brought some relief. The area was wet, sore, and swollen. Alternately, green clay and German chamomile were used, which calmed down the inflammation and eventually cleared it up. We were able to keep the area clear for months by using zoopharmacognosy. Amazing!

During various phone calls to the breeders and while visiting Hagrid at their kennels, I'd requested information about him. Nothing had been mentioned, except to advise I use Aloe Vera gel to treat a couple of spots under his chin, he liked his tummy rubbed, and that he was a 'lazy' dog. More questions were raised as the food provided was poor quality and wasn't sustaining him. The little background information that was offered, together with poor quality food, led me to wonder what the truth really was.

The vet prescribed various medications including some antimicrobial skin cleanser to put on and around his face and neck area. After a couple of days of administering it, Hagrid began to growl at me when I came close. So what could I do now? Go with what the vet prescribed or try something else?

Sometimes carers can take the easy path without thinking things through. Incorporating preventative strategies may mean medication can be avoided, because the dog is in a healthier position all round.

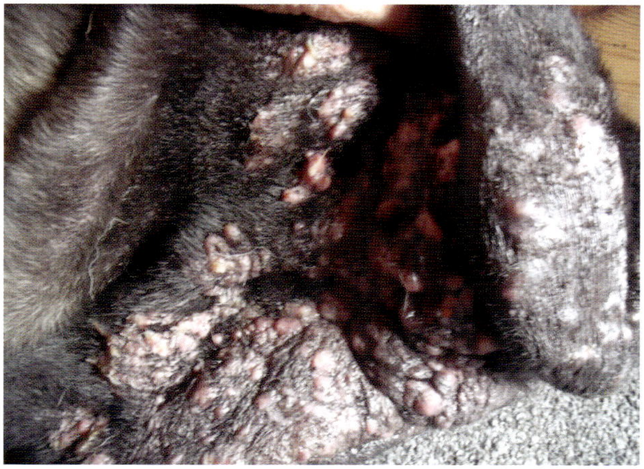

Underneath Hagrid's fur was inflamed skin that oozed and bled. The worst part was the irritation. It was most frustrating for him in the evening, and if the central heating was on. This photo was taken quite early on, about a year after he joined us.

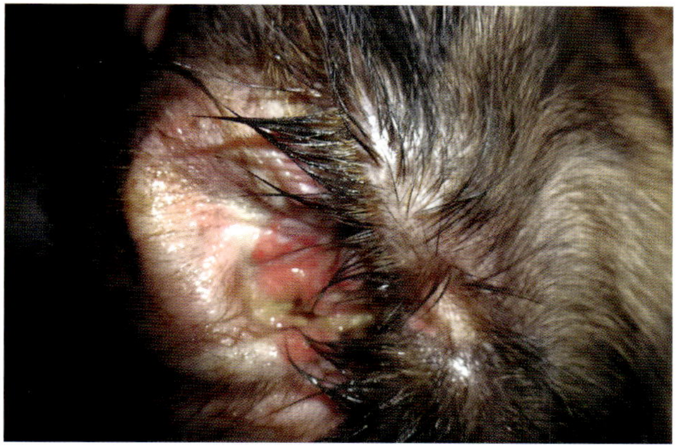

Hagrid's ears, probably at their worst. Although many veterinary preparations were used, it seemed that nothing worked long-term. It was a case of managing the symptoms. Green clay was used regularly; this soothed and helped sustain them intermittently while we worked on improving his internal state too. The idea was to work on building his internal health, whilst treating the topical symptoms.

While vets have incredible knowledge, they don't live with us or know our dogs to the extent that we do. It can be a more effective treatment if we can combine their knowledge with our understanding of our dogs and their lives. It's a collaborative relationship that requires us all, in different aspects of our dogs' lives, to try to work out what's best. It was great that Hagrid was able to communicate with me, and so it was my job to listen, understand and gain his trust. For whatever reason, he didn't like or want the medication, so I respected his request and backed off. Instead I decided to explore alternatives that he could tolerate, that wouldn't make him react in a defensive way.

When starting to respect a dog's signs, in the way that you would want your own boundaries and feelings to be listened to, you can start to establish trust. They know that they can rely on their carer not to push them into compromising situations they're uncomfortable with, and that when they communicate something, they will be listened to.

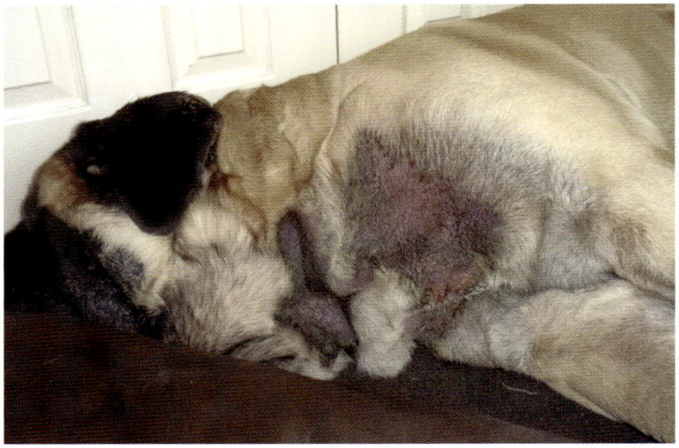

Under skin folds on Hagrid's neck. In this picture it's possible to see where and why a harness or a collar would irritate and why both were used at different times with the aim to prevent contact with the sore skin. With Hagrid's collar, I extended it so it was oversized then attached a few small stones to it, weighing it down so that the clip the lead was attached to stayed on top. With thoughtful handling, it worked so there was minimal contact at the front of his neck. I was careful to follow behind him on walks as much as possible.

We were always working on Hagrid's health issues, trying to improve the quality of his life through careful handling and management, experiences, diet, and exercise, as well as with relationships to people and animals. Despite this, at several periods in his life he was critically ill and I'd been advised on a number of occasions that he wouldn't live for much longer.

My previous Mastiff, Kaos, had died at the age of just five years, and I didn't anticipate that Hagrid would even reach that. Amazingly, Hagrid lived to eight and a half! In this time, he enjoyed an enriched life, and I believe he did *incredibly* well to achieve that longevity.

Visible symptoms of a much deeper problem

Dogs are like humans: if they're healthy on the inside, it shows on the outside, as in healthy skin, hair and eyes.

During one particularly difficult phase in Hagrid's life – before we'd come across zoopharmacognosy (see side panel) – he was having regular bouts of chronic poo in the night. I dreaded coming downstairs every day, being greeted by the terrible smell and what looked like projective poo filling my office. Can you imagine Hagrid's desperation and how he must have felt? He'd never been scolded for soiling in our house but at this stage he wasn't able to communicate with us.

Over time, Hagrid learned to ask to go out into the garden to go to the toilet, but back then he was still lacking the confidence to communicate.

For all of us, having the confidence to ask takes time for trust to develop. Looking back, I realise just how much zoopharmacognosy improved Hagrid's life. He was a transformed dog in his last three and a half years, in some ways getting healthier as he aged. How great was that?

Eighteen months before he developed brain problems he looked the best he ever had, with strong well-developed muscles, a coat that was in good, healthy condition, skin that had never been better, with no more pustules, no more clearing his throat, the lumps in his neck had long gone, and the bleeding and diarrhoea had disappeared. In part because of this, Hagrid's behaviour had improved too, hardly paying any attention to people as they walked by us while out on walks.

He was content and happy.

About zoopharmacognosy

Briefly, zoopharmacognosy (or self-selection) is a process where an animal is subtly and gently offered a variety of oils, compounds or herbs that they can choose from what they instinctively know they need for their own healing. It's based on the idea that the body recognises what's required to be in balance, and this translates into their choices from the selection offered. It's both an indicator of components required for health benefits, and a therapy in itself, with them being able to access appropriate substances they need.

Self-selection will be explained in more detail later. After using it for a period of time, however, Hagrid's skin mostly became clear of inflammation. His ears remained an intermittent, ongoing concern, and part of the skin under his neck and chest had flare-ups now and then. These were treated and kept under control through zoopharmacognosy, both internally and externally/topically.

CHAPTER 7

Walks

A walk's a walk, right? We do it every day, so how is it possible to write so many words about it?

The reason I've chosen to include a few thoughts here is that there is a significant difference between what is of interest to a dog and what is of interest to a human.

Imagine for a moment you are a dog, whose main daily adventure is a walk. Now that you have the sense of smell, and freedom from all material worries and concerns that a dog enjoys, wouldn't you want to spend the time exploring every part of your environment - once, maybe twice a day for some dogs? The time isn't important, it's what you do in that time and having one quality, fulfilling walk (or two shorter ones) a day can be satisfying.

Imagine enjoying a hobby, something that absorbs your attention, is stimulating and gives a sense of accomplishment. Doesn't it feel gratifying when that's something you have spent time over?

Walks are a chance to have individual time with my dogs; we can be together and connected. Very occasionally we all go out at once, which works well when there are handlers for each dog and each of them has the space they need. When dogs become used to the concept of making choices I'm amazed by their clever decisions, and the things they teach me daily. One of ours usually prefers to be separate from the others on walks, choosing to go in a totally different direction. Fortunately, she can have this luxury. It's interesting to see them make decisions like this.

I was grateful to Hagrid's previous owners for several reasons, some of which I've talked about: the most obvious of course is that they were happy for him to come and live with us! They'd been open and available for my other dog Jaffa and Hagrid to be walked around their field on the two occasions we'd visited. Plus, he hadn't been over-exercised, which in my experience, quite a few dogs are. He hadn't had a ball or other toys thrown for him to chase and catch, which many dogs do on their walks.

Hagrid was accustomed to wandering around in their field with the other dogs he'd lived with. I was told he didn't move about much and was 'lazy' but if you or I had health problems and were a bully's victim, how much would we want to move around and risk being targeted?

At first, walks must have seemed alien to Hagrid, having never been on one before. I wondered what he thought. When I'd asked where the breeders walked their dogs, they looked puzzled and said they didn't walk them because they had their own field. Having reflected on this, I could appreciate that walking twenty or more dogs would not be easy, especially when eleven of them were Mastiffs! It could've taken all day. However, I know people who walk the same number of dogs daily, albeit less sizeable ones, in small groups. This may not always be ideal for all of the dogs, and a close eye has to be taken on each one and their changing needs to ensure they're comfortable in the group setting.

The first time we walked Hagrid he just walked and walked, at the end of an eight metre lead, without any interaction with his surroundings or looking back at us. This indicated to me that he was an uncomfortable dog who, for whatever reason, felt unable to trust. Also, he was probably worried and unfamiliar with being walked in a new place.

To start with, I kept walks short; usually 5 -15 minutes at a time depending on how he seemed. We stuck to one place in the beginning, so he could develop familiarity with that particular environment, which was suitable for many reasons; quiet, not much going on, open space to be able to see, and not too populated. Open spaces don't suit all dogs.

However the first few metres at the start wasn't ideal for him because it was quite a confined space, although it might be more suitable for some dogs, but it created the least amount of fuss. We'd go at quiet times of the day to minimise bumping into anyone coming out of their houses. After all, neither of us knew what to expect from interactions with people or animals. Most people would not have described what we did as 'going for a walk'. It began to make a difference, however.

I remember one particular stroll when we reached the field closest to our house. Hagrid had just become more aware of his environment and was sniffing around. On entering the field, he had a sniff, a wee and like a spring lamb almost skipped along for a second or two. He was happy, showing the lovely dog he was, and we both felt the positive energy in that. It was springtime in Hagrid's new life. The scared dog we'd adopted was slowly trusting and embracing life.

Dogs can lack confidence, not feel secure enough to wee and/or poo on walks, and sometimes this can happen in the privacy of their own gardens.

Insecurity came out for Hagrid as not lifting his leg, but at this point he felt relaxed enough to be able to, and I was so happy when he felt comfortable enough to do that.

After a couple of months, I began to take him out in the van, which he liked. We found quiet places to go with him, because then going for a walk was enough in itself without the added distractions of people, dogs, traffic and other animals. He wasn't in the position to sniff properly at first because of being worried, so we kept these sessions short, going back to our base point. It was important that these introductions were at his pace, in other words at a pace that didn't overwhelm or stress him too much, so he could see new things in a positive light, without causing any issues through negative associations.

Equipment

Hagrid was limited by a few health issues, despite his young age. I was well aware of the effect of over-exercise and exposing a dog to too many new, stimulating environments that could impact on his wellness. For walks, Hagrid always wore a soft fleece harness or a loosely fitting wide collar, depending on the current condition of his skin and which piece of equipment made the least contact on affected areas. Because he'd been used to a collar while with the breeders, going slowly when wearing a harness was necessary.

Clipped onto the collar was a long line. I use various lengths and that is determined by which dog I'm with; usually five or eight metres for my larger dogs. These leads are suitable for the different areas each walk requires. You'll read a lot about the importance of using a long lead. I think the majority of dogs may benefit by being walked on one provided they are handled in a nurturing, sensitive and compassionate way. This requires thought and care as the lead glides gently through one hand using a light pressure so the dog and handler feel a supportive connection between one another. It's a little like holding someone's hand lightly. When the dog slows and stops to sniff, the handler has a chance to walk towards them and the other hand gathers up the lead in loops and then out again as the dog moves off. Going closer involves the person walking their hands down the lead toward the dog, avoiding mishandling in pulling the dog back to them.

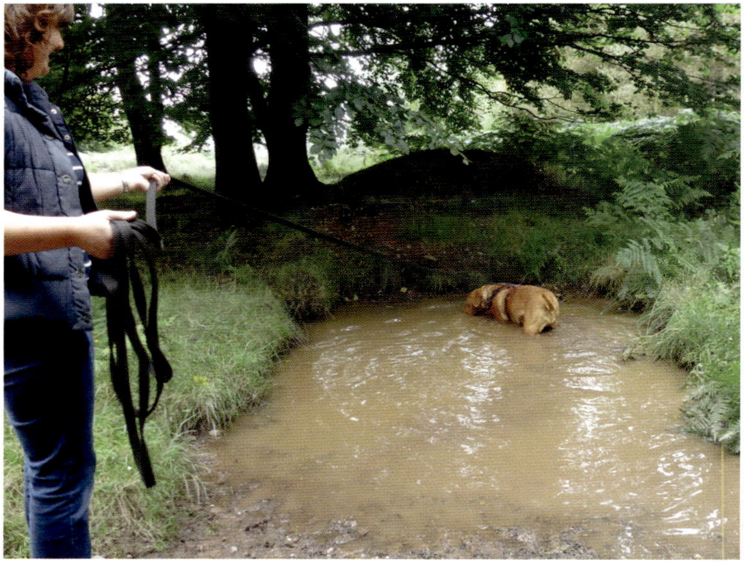

Hannah's dog, Nessa, wades into a large muddy puddle and Hannah supports her choice. The long line ensures that the dog has a connection to the handler, and that she's kept safe around anything that might appear.

Slight movements on the lead can mean a dog is interrupted, sometimes triggering them to do something, maybe react, especially if too close. Imagine how you feel when interrupted in the middle of doing something, especially if it happens several times; it may provoke a reaction in you. Being aware of the small movements we make on the lead, how a dog might feel and noticing his response is quite enlightening; then it's possible to be mindful and better placed to give them a good feeling from the walk.

The handler offers choices, within the range of the lead, so the dog can be safe and gain a comfortable and suitable distance to be able to explore and sniff in peace.

The above gives a brief insight into using a long lead, but there's far more to it than meets the eye. Being taught to use a long line effectively makes so much difference to the way a dog behaves, and if done smoothly, this gives them an easy experience with minimal impact on their walk. It's also a great way to get to know more about the dog. Please look up Sheila Harper for more information - details can be found at the back of the book.

A woven fabric lead of five metres or more, depending on the dog's needs, offers the experience of a tactile two-way connection with which both dog and carer can work. The idea is that long lines are used in a way that has as little impact on the dog and their walk as possible, while maintaining communication with, and a safe boundary for, them.

With a long line, it's possible to influence a dog gently so that he can think of an alternative option, rather than having to pull back against him and create tension. Taking this approach means it's possible to subtly guide him to a more suitable environment, which may limit pulling, provided time is given to process the information.

> You'll see from the photo opposite that long lines are a fixed length, not to be confused with an extendable lead, used so that the length is constantly adapted to match what is needed in the situation.

By gradually increasing a little pressure on the lead, it's a message that the lead is coming to the end so the stop happens smoothly and not suddenly. Then he has the option to decide what to do next. This demonstrates just one way to use a long line with empathy.

Extendable leads

For some people, using extendable leads may be necessary in certain circumstances, although I always encourage clients to become familiar with using a long line so they can help their dog develop skills. Extendable leads are quite definite; it's either stop or go, with barely anything in between. The handler may try to stop gently, although the dog will feel a jolt as the brake is applied, with no idea when it's going to happen. The stop comes suddenly and without warning, which can be a shock, especially if they were excited and moving quickly.

If the sudden halt happens when they're worried about something they are looking at, the negative experience could reinforce anxiety, and they may be more concerned the next time they encounter it. Pain or shock at the time of encountering a specific object, person or animal can be associated with what they're seeing, creating uncertainty and unease.

The noise as the winder mechanism kicks in can be quite distressing for some dogs; again another trigger to reinforce associations with worrying encounters. Sound-sensitive and nervous dogs are particularly vulnerable and may become reactive to the noises from the lead.

Aside from this, there are purely safety considerations. People and dogs have been tangled up in extendable leads, and because it's quite a thin wire, have been injured. This is especially likely if the dog is excitable and inclined to suddenly pull.

My dog pulls – why is this?

A lot of people, including myself, wonder why their dog is pulling.

My dogs rarely do what I'd call 'pull', but it was a different story not so long ago. Occasionally there are situations that crop up when they feel the need to speed up, go further than the long line allows, or beyond the limit I apply for them. I look to see what is happening to cause this but 'pulling' is a good way for a dog to make their feelings clear to me, which I encourage and I find it useful information. Pulling is a way a dog expresses what's going on within them at the time; how they feel.

I have learnt to turn things around so that they teach me to be much more observant. When they aren't pulling, just ambling along, stopping to sniff at this and that, I take notice what is going on - the conditions, as all of these affect a dog's degree of pulling. By that I mean:

Where are we?

In a quiet area; at a distance from other dogs and people; in a park; walking along a street.

Who is with me?

Children; other adults; other animals.

What's in the vicinity?

Is there traffic nearby? It can cause some dogs to move faster. Are we in an open or enclosed space with coverage? Trees, bushes, shrubs etc. Is it open for me and covered for the dogs? What wildlife is likely to live there? What is the weather like?

What can my dogs see, hear and smell?

I may not know the answer to that.

Space

Often dogs need to gain adequate space from the handler to feel comfortable, just as we need space from others to feel at ease. Using a long line allows dogs to have this choice in many situations, limiting the need to pull.

Further into my investigation I think about whether anything happened on the way to the destination, because sensory factors can accumulate for some dogs, and the intensity comes out as pulling or in unwanted behaviours, which are just the dog's way of communicating. Some have expectations on regular routes that can cause them to be excited, pulling in anticipation of reaching a destination such as the park where their lead is often unclipped. I also look back to what the previous few hours and days were like before we came out to see if they've had a particularly calm time at home with not much happening or if there have been numerous visitors, postmen, deliveries, or whether the dogs encountered a particularly busy week, with long walks, trips here and there, and so on. Are they in good health or could something be going on for them? All of these factors will impact on the way dogs behave on their walks.

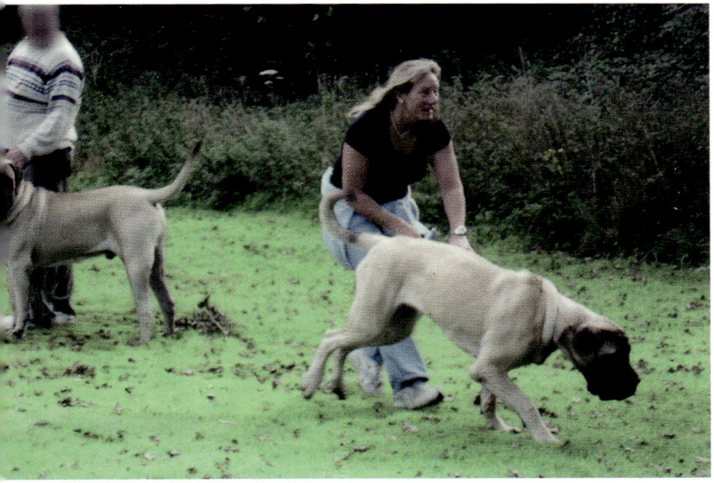

One reason a dog will pull. I've used this photo – also used in my 'Understanding the Silent Communication of Dogs' book – because back in those days Kaos had to use strong language for me to listen, accept and respond to her feelings. Here she is pulling me away from a situation she'd been faced with before, and didn't want to go through again. Dogs are likely to show subtle language before reaching this stage, although if it's been ignored often enough, they may go straight to pulling. It's about tuning into their communication, considering how it is for them and not just blindly doing what we want.

I find that by noticing and being inquisitive, I set the scene for further peaceful walks that my dogs relish. So by looking at what has contributed to them sauntering and sniffing means I find ways to recreate that on future walks by replicating the conditions.

Dogs pull for all kinds of reasons and often we can do something about it by looking at what's happening (or not happening) when they can just potter around, taking time to sniff at this and that. I need to mention here that a suitable environment, and again a longer lead/line, gives them space needed to settle down and sniff so they don't have to pull. A dog will often speed up because he doesn't have enough space from the handler.

Leads are usually manufactured for peoples' convenience, and are too short for dogs. We've been conditioned to have a dog close to us and under control.

Walking dogs together

Many dogs enjoy the company of another dog on a walk but some dogs struggle with this. I have given a lot of time to observing and thinking about what it might be like for a dog to be walked with other dogs.

When Colin and I walk our dogs together, we might separate and meet up at various points along the way depending on what each dog communicates, so that they spend some time together, and some apart. As with ours, tension can build the longer the walk continues. They can have very different needs and walking them separately is a great way to meet these. Otherwise, a dog is likely to struggle because he has to be with the group and keep up. It's hard for them to be different or show vulnerability. Have you ever been with someone who is fitter and gone along with them to please them, pushing yourself? This is often how it is for dogs. The number and duration of walks a dog has vary according to each one's needs and is dependent on age, health, breed and hormones too.

Walking dogs individually means that it's possible to observe, get to know their preferences and notice changes as the walk progresses. When they're with another dog, it's easier for them to become tired for example, and then when signals are spotted, it's often too late to do something. Dogs living with other dogs will undoubtedly need to be alone at some point. This will be for all kinds of reasons, and having time when they are living as individuals in their own right is healthy and a way to develop self-assurance. Done appropriately for each one, being apart inside the house at certain times, as well as separate on some walks, gives them the best chance of a healthy relationship with one another.

Meeting other dogs on walks

Giving Hagrid special time on walks was wonderful. We met other dogs when he was confident and well enough to deal with them. Initially, he invaded other dogs' space, as he'd done when first meeting Jaffa. Usually though, after a sniff, it was okay to move on without further interest. As I put in boundaries to prevent the intrusion, he gradually learned to respect their space and needs. Many dogs are put off and can of course be quite fearful of one as big as him. Hagrid also had a strong smell that didn't help matters. I learned dogs could be afraid of ones who are unwell, meaning quite a few would bark at him, which wasn't nice for either animal. Hagrid didn't like being barked at, and would want to go home straight away if it happened. No dog likes having to bark or being barked at.

We'd walk Jaffa and Hagrid together now and then. Being with Jaffa outside gave Hagrid confidence. She was confident on walks and around most dogs, but I'd still give her help when she needed it, not just leave her to her own devices. No matter how well adjusted, all dogs need some support and guidance from time to time in the complex world they share with us. Seeing one or two friendly dogs now and then on a walk is probably enough for most balanced dogs.

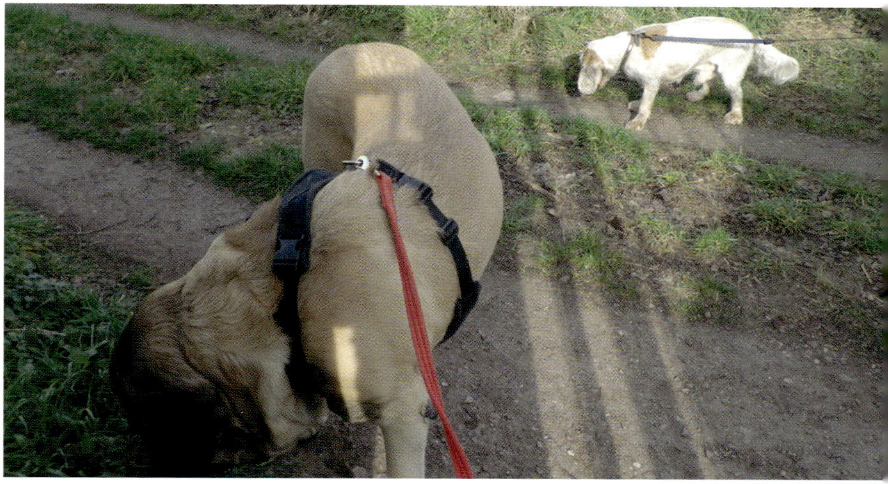

Hagrid was walking with one of his friends, a spaniel called Coley. Both were introduced over several months, at a distance at first, following each other's smell before actually seeing each other. Then they'd catch glimpses of the other. On another walk they might be a little closer and so on. One day Coley chose to come closer to Hagrid, once he trusted his communication would be respected and he'd be able to move away when he decided to. It still took a few more walks before he made the decision he'd like to go and meet Hagrid up close. Their walks were calm, sniffing around together and just enjoying each other's company. That's how dogs often choose to do things when they have a say in it; calmly being together, then parting and doing their own thing.

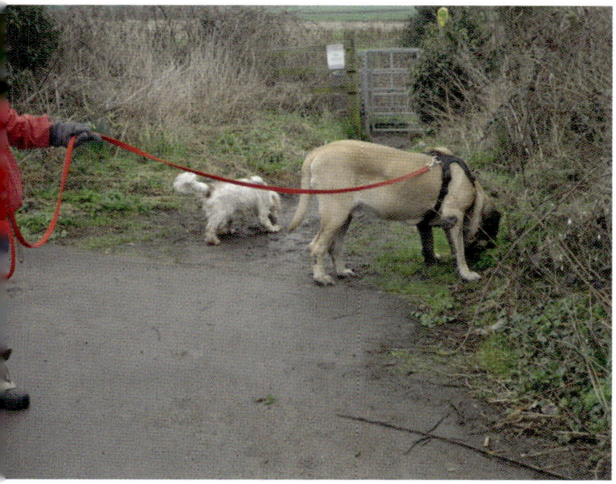

Note Hagrid's curved body language near Coley, deflecting his attention away from him and helping Coley to feel more relaxed as opposed to a more intense direct interaction.

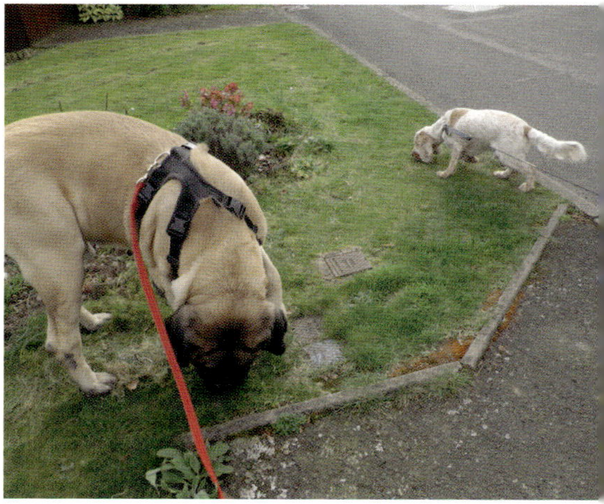

Hagrid and other animals

Hagrid was used to being around other animals; namely pigs and goats. But in many ways he hadn't been spoiled with over-socialisation. For him, mixing with them appeared to happen in a natural, informal and relaxed way: they were there and that was that, just another part of life.

At first they interacted at a large distance, where he could watch for a little while without reacting. Often this natural and comfortable approach to socialisation is better than making a point or big issue of them meeting and being too close too soon.

It's important to know that there can be undercurrents of communication that go unnoticed in these circumstances. In Hagrid's case, there was bullying that most probably started long before anyone noticed, and can be subtle. We only need to think of how it is for humans who are bullied to get a sense of how it may be for an animal.

I must mention here that when people talk about dogs bullying or intimidating other animals, the negative terms involved aren't really helpful as they can create resentment, whereas the best approach to these kind of behaviours is to understand and empathise with the perpetrator and go from there. Having unfavourable feelings towards a dog that is already going to have strong negativity in its emotions, if it's bullying another, only furthers a cycle of bad feeling without resolving it.

Something is causing that behaviour to happen, and laying blame can aggravate the situation. Hagrid's behaviour at the time would indicate that he was worried or feeling some kind of insecurity, just as people do. I was able to empathise with him, which softened my feelings and made it possible to make a few changes before he felt the need to intimidate. This was more productive and helps a victim more than anything. Blaming and punishing is an adverse reaction; understanding and being observant sets the scene for change, moving forward.

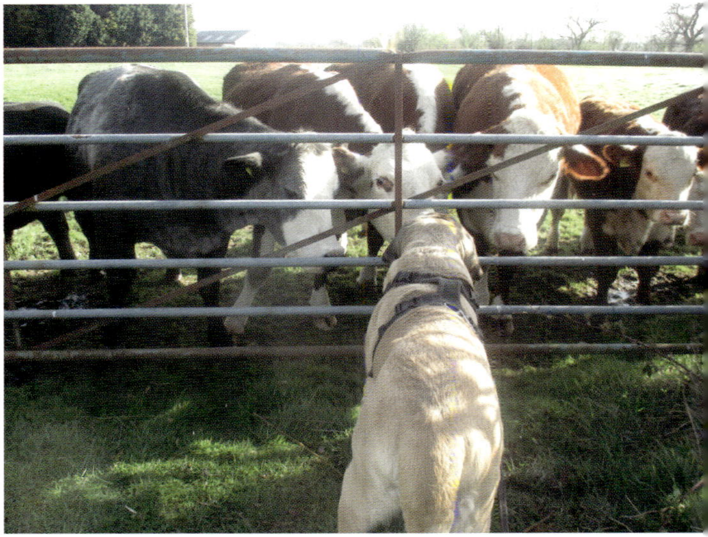

Hagrid and these cows met frequently. They'd come across the field to see him as he rested at the gateway. A beautiful relationship.

Sometimes when dogs live together, there can be elements of coercion for survival's sake, and this can be so subtle that we miss it. When a dog is – or has been – bullied, or shows insecure behaviours that threaten others, they can go on to exhibit what they've learnt. We knew Hagrid had been threatened from at least one other dog in his previous home, and this was one of the reasons he came to live with us.

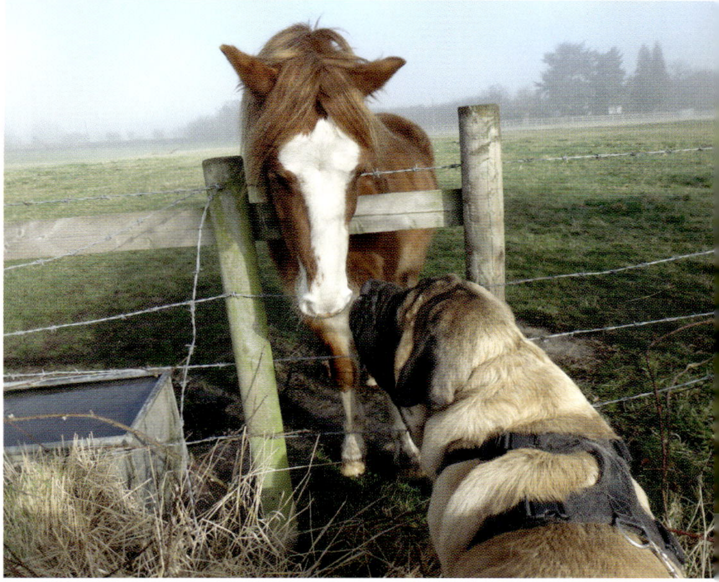

There were also horses we'd meet regularly. Hagrid would decide which way to walk and chose to visit them sometimes. The young horse always came to visit him, sometimes accompanied by an older horse and Hagrid was gentle as they sniffed each other. At times his smell put the horses off from coming too close.

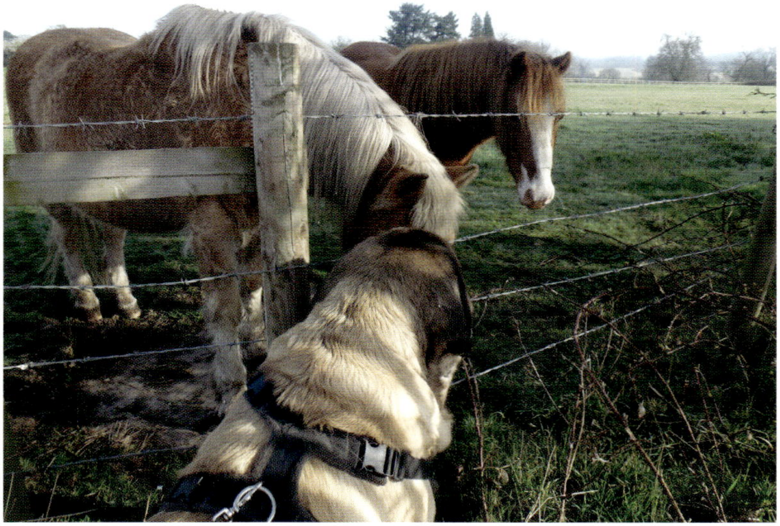

Learning to manage people on walks

Where we lived, our neighbours were wonderful and very understanding. When I called round to ask each of them to just get on with whatever they were doing if ever they saw me out with Hagrid, that's what they did, and it helped him immensely. At first, he'd see someone on their drive carrying on with their daily chores and he'd stop, look and sniff, and I'd wait until he was ready to come with me. Sometimes I felt embarrassed at the length of time we stood there while he watched. It seemed like a long time; it was, but doing that a few times helped Hagrid build a positive, unobtrusive picture of humans.

In time, it wasn't as much of an issue. He could see them, look, be interested and carry on if they continued with their business. It did take him time because, after all, he was Hagrid and so took that extra time to process information.

Asking people to give us space and leave Hagrid alone didn't always work. At times it wasn't possible to move him out of a situation without him becoming suspicious, so I honed my skills in distracting people who approached by asking them about themselves, if it was too rude to ignore someone. This took the focus off Hagrid and allowed him to settle. With the long lead he was able to sniff at nearby smells that were of interest. Using my body, I could position myself to make challenging situations easier for him while also keeping an eye on him to see how he was doing.

Completely avoiding encounters was also needed sometimes, together with learning to manage situations effectively. One tool I learned if I saw someone coming was to use my body language to deflect attention away from them. For example, I would put my focus on what Hagrid was sniffing, which would keep him occupied. Dogs can pick up on which direction we're looking and if our breathing patterns change, which is likely to happen when we're concerned about something. They are attuned to our emotional state often before we are!

The tactics I used depended on the situation. I would use the long line as a tool for matching my approach with the environment. When on a pavement along a road, the lead could be gently gathered in to a shorter length by walking my hands down it toward the dog. As he wandered down driveways, or the pathway widened or narrowed, the lead was adjusted accordingly. This is working with a dog in the environment, to allow for what is going on.

Another useful tool was to train myself not to panic and rush Hagrid along, even if something we encountered might be a potential problem. When I learned to do that, I was often surprised to find everything was actually fine, which didn't mean I put Hagrid into a situation he found difficult just because he'd dealt with it before. It showed what stage we were at in his development and gave me confidence that being calm, whatever the outcome, was more effective.

First and foremost, training *myself* to respond calmly to situations really benefitted Hagrid because, as mentioned earlier, dogs intuitively pick up on our mood. Consequently, they're more likely to react and think something must be really worrying if we do. By remaining calm, we can reduce a dog's anxiety.

More and more, I learned that being relaxed and grounded is a positive place from which to respond, for any dog and scenario. It enabled me to observe, and made it easier to deal with anything that arose.

For the last few years of Hagrid's life he was able to deal well with the people we met. I'd made sure Hagrid had many positive non-events where people had just walked past as they do with other dogs. I also asked people to leave him alone and not stroke him.

On the odd occasion when someone didn't listen, or they appeared too quickly to ask, Hagrid had been fine. By fine I mean that he'd dealt with it, although he wasn't especially happy, but he managed. This didn't mean I wanted anyone to approach him just because he'd be fine. But the more he was able to be part of everyday life without having attention drawn to him, the more he learnt it was okay and able to accept people passing by.

Challenging situations do arise – that's part of life – it's what we do or don't do that counts. Being at ease helps any other parties who may be involved and positively influences the eventual outcome.

Exploring the neighbourhood

Once he was settled on walks, I slowly began to increase the areas we visited. There were two or three basic regular walking routes with which he was familiar. In total, we had about six to eight routes of varying lengths that were suitable at different times of the year. For example on hotter days, shady trails that took us near the river were preferable to a farmyard walk, which was open and giving very little shade. Bales of hay in nearby fields offered so much interest to Hagrid at certain times of the year, so I'd try to take him there, and he became fully absorbed in what had been around them.

These considerations and others are decisions that can be made for most dogs on all of their walks. I make choices on where to go for each of mine, dependent on their needs, how they are on the day, the time of year, wildlife that may be around, and how much time is available. I'd also think about the challenge of any particular walk; what had been going on for them in the previous few days, the time of day, weather, length of walk and so on. These are just some of the thoughts upon which our walks were based.

During winter months when the weather was very wet and people tended to be inside, there was an opportunity for walks that involved narrower pavements on the way to a local field, but when the weather was fine, it wasn't an option. At those times, driving a short way from the house provided more opportunities, and we used them as often as we could.

Hagrid's experiences grew over the years, and for the last two or three he was able to have town walks at times when most people would be in bed, usually early on a Sunday morning or at other quiet times such as bank holidays. Those walks were very enriching for him; one street walk in particular was interesting. Along this row of shops there were two hairdressers, a butcher's shop, a Chinese takeaway, a launderette, a cake and sandwich shop, a betting office and an off licence.

There were several alluring points for a dog here. Three circular plant tubs which other dogs regularly weed up, discarded bits of food and rubbish, the doormat outside the butchers, and the back of the shops. Hagrid had a routine of thoroughly sniffing the mat at the butcher's, weeing up the bin and flower tubs close to the shop, sniffing the walls, and looking into bins. Behind the row of shops there were often new objects to be explored. As he became less able to walk the short way from our house to these shops, only a few hundred metres away, I would drive him there. Towards the end of his life I found suitable areas like this to walk him, adapting to his changing needs, making sure there was something engaging as he came out of the van.

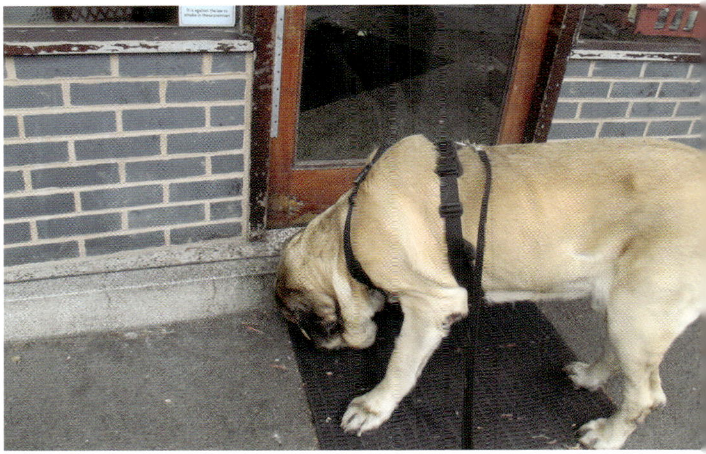

The doormat outside the butcher's shop gave Hagrid many happy moments while he inhaled the smells.

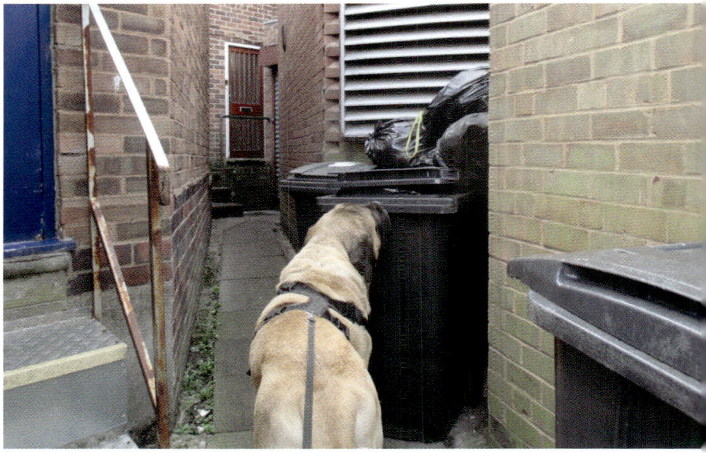

Behind the bread shop. Hagrid was a regular visitor to the bins, which he always sniffed at his leisure. He never tried to pull the bags out, although he could have done. This was enough and he was satisfied. I've found gradually trusting my dogs is a great way to allow natural behaviours and avoid any tensioned situations which can create unhealthy obsessions, particularly with food.

The pavement outside the shops was wide and people occasionally walked past as Hagrid enjoyed the smells. In all the years we came here, we encountered just a handful of dogs on these early Sunday morning/bank holiday excursions. Bins and flower tubs acted as barriers to break up any direct interactions, which helped.

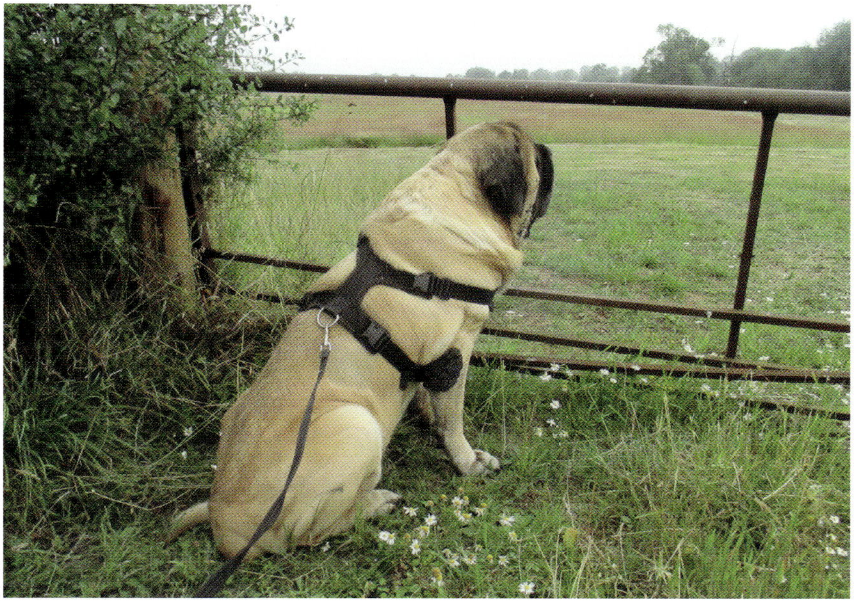

Again, the walk was relatively short, but it offered Hagrid so much stimulation. We'd often see horses, donkeys, sheep and alpacas in the fields close by.

Other pavements didn't offer the space Hagrid needed; they were too narrow to comfortably walk along and not an ideal place for dogs to pass. I like to make sure mine have the space with which they feel at ease when walking along pavements, so try to give them as much room from others as possible. This usually means crossing the road. For some there needs to be much more distance. Not all have been comfortable being by roads, so walks are tailored to suit the individual.

People like to follow paths but it's possible to adjust and move off them to give a dog some choices and exploration time. This depends on my dogs' experiences and can steadily enable them to develop their curiosity when the moment is right.

Information gathering

Sniffing out items of interest is how dogs gather information. They gain confidence in their surroundings and knowledge about the world around them; other dogs, people and animals who've been in the area, which can include their age, gender, health, and emotional well-being. A dog will know how recent the smells are and make decisions about them, given the chance. I like to notice what they choose to do after sniffing certain smells. When Kuzu was on one particular walk, he suddenly became very intent on tracking a scent, to an extent that I'd never seen before. It reached the point that he pulled so much because he was a strong dog, that the walk became unenjoyable for both of us. I shortened the lead and took him home to give him chance to calm down and ease his frustrations. He was exhausted, but the walk had only lasted about ten minutes. I later discovered that a couple of hours before, a bitch in season had been in the area.

We can usually influence their decisions and reactions to these things if we need to; many will need help initially. It's unfair to let them do what they want all the time, it requires a fair balance. An example is the situation mentioned above. Naturally, it wouldn't be appropriate for Kuzu to find the bitch that was on heat, so instead we needed a boundary in the form of a shortened lead and shorter walk.

Outside, there's the opportunity to leave messages for other dogs and occasionally meet one or two that they feel totally at ease with, providing they have the skills to deal with meetings. Seeing others and gradually getting to know them is important and at times, for some, meeting up with one another can be fulfilling and enhance a walk.

Sharing part of the walk with another dog is something many of them enjoy, and it's crucial to understand their communication to know they're happy with each other. Using a long line ensures they have a safe choice and are supported; without one they're much more vulnerable.

From the beginning, dogs are not taught how to be around other dogs, and are regularly left to their own devices. Their communication is so quick that it's difficult for people to comprehend. Without being able to have a break, they are often left together for way too long, and it's more likely than not that one dog struggles. This is common, but of course not always the case. To leave their carer or to avoid a dog with whom they're walking takes a brave and confident dog. Quite a few aren't able to do this, so need us to understand their communication.

When they have come too close to other dogs it's harder for them to express their feelings adequately and be acknowledged. Anxiety may be present by this point, and then it's harder for them to communicate with us, particularly if both become anxious. Just think about the challenges humans face when trying to express their apprehensions with someone who is anxious, or when two angry people are attempting to be heard! The same principle applies: space and a relaxed approach can do wonders for our ability to think, assess and make better choices.

Dogs meeting each other is something quite a few people focus on, but it's the journey that's important. Consider how necessary it is to feel that you have communicated and left messages for your fellow humans. Making friends usually happens over time, although people meet others every day. If they have the skills they can choose to come away when they want, or make excuses out of politeness, etc. It can be similar for dogs, but some may lack those skills, then it can become intense, and that's when one (both, really) can suffer.

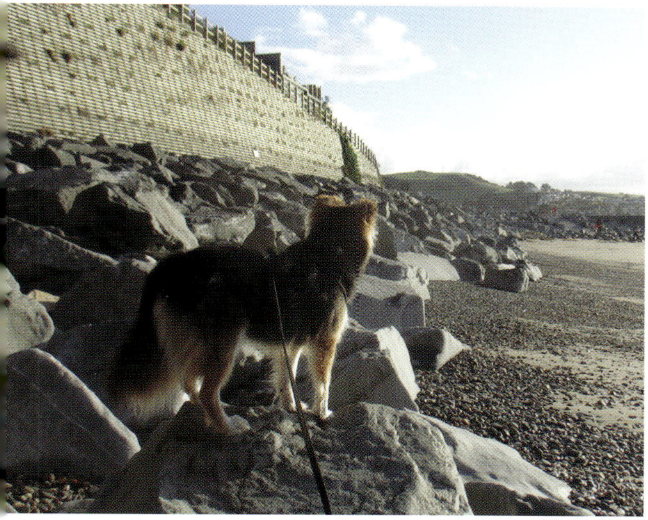

Pogo in one of her favourite spots, enjoying an early morning walk. She's taking some time to watch someone and their dog at the far end of the beach, before moving on.

Barking

When Hagrid's confidence had grown, he entered a stage of barking at people. On one occasion, I asked a man who was standing where we intended to go if he'd mind looking the other way as we walked past him. Another option would have been to go back, which I knew Hagrid wouldn't be able to do at that point, because of being scared of this man and freezing on the spot. Many dogs freeze with fear and can't move when they're worried and too close to something.

I decided that co-operation was the best way to deal with this. Hagrid's barking was an advance on his previous coping behaviour: slithering along the ground. It meant that he felt more confident to react, which was better, in the grand scheme of his emotional well-being, than not reacting at all. The lovely man was so helpful, did as I asked, and because he'd been willing to help us it made it so much easier for Hagrid to walk past him. This was another great step forward in trusting people. As we passed, I thanked him for his co-operation as I was really grateful he worked with us. It's important to thank people for their helpfulness. A good, positive, outcome – for everyone! We saw the man a few times and the non-event became easier for all of us.

Most dogs attract attention and big ones usually attract a lot. They rarely want this from strangers; not the way it often happens anyway. None of my dogs enjoy people they don't know coming up to them and Hagrid really didn't. People might obviously be quite surprised when they see a big dog and, when surprised, it's common to stop and stare. I've noticed some talk to the dog and handler, maintain full eye contact with the dog and even reach out to touch them. All this attention creates a static situation that dogs usually find difficult and frustrating, especially the longer the focus continues. This is particularly the case when it's someone they don't know and sometimes even when they do. If the dog has the choice to approach or not and people keep their hands to themselves, that generally makes it a little easier for them. There are plenty, however, who receive attention now and then and deal with it, but generally, when you're a Mastiff you create a reaction like this from people everywhere you go. I also saw that Hagrid didn't bark at people who carried on with whatever they were doing, rather than giving us attention.

Imagine for a moment being the centre of attention when you're least expecting it. How would that feel? You might feel nervous, embarrassed, shy and so on. Notice the kind of reactions young children have. It's understandable that when people stop and stare, they might be barked at by a dog who doesn't know why they're staring. This can be quite intimidating for both.

Eventually, a dog might even begin to bark at the sight of a person because of the fear of what might come next. If the dog's lower-level communication signals aren't listened to, naturally they would escalate their language, and might start to become animated, jump up, bark, growl or snap at people.

Loss of confidence

Lack of confidence on walks needs to be assessed, especially if it's a regular occurrence. Many behaviour problems can begin because there's an underlying health issue that hasn't yet been detected. Other points can be considered; the dog feels insecure with their surroundings, which may be unsuitable. Maybe the dog needs shorter walks, certain smells put them off going that way, or they require a more suitable place, for example. I know for my dogs that being on a long line helps their confidence. Pogo knows when she'd like to be on her lead; some dogs get to know it offers security and support.

At times Hagrid lost confidence and, when it happened, if I looked back to other times we were in that area, I could usually remember an incident such as being barked at.

That was enough to put him off going somewhere. Being listened to if he was showing signs he didn't want to be there, giving the time he needed to think and adjust, was so important. Many dogs could benefit from this kind of help and support. Walking away and leaving them to deal with it is going to make a dog less confident and worry more on walks and is hurtful to see one struggle so much. Encouragement could work for Hagrid and be suitable at times, but unsuitable at others. We'd go back a few months later then surprisingly it would be fine. For dogs that have been forced in the past, are in pain, uncomfortable, fearful and so on, it's best to seek advice from the vet. The key is understanding the individual dog and looking at the context.

On occasions when Hagrid couldn't cope, we'd go to other places he knew well. Later it would be different and no longer a problem for him. But what matters is that we tried other options, gave him time, didn't force him and Hagrid was happy with that. Incidentally, Pogo is easily put off an area by smells of some dogs that are walked there, without seeing them. Luckily, when this happens she is given other routes to choose from.

Sitting on walks

A favourite walk of Hagrid's was along a wide grassy track with hedges and rabbit burrows on either side. He'd sit at various points, either at the end or halfway through. One way to describe these moments is as if he were appreciating the time, smells and what was going on. I also liked just being with him, together in the calm and peace of nature. Hagrid would sit and sniff until he'd had enough, and sometimes a smell would entice him to get up and investigate what had wafted his way. There was usually something worth getting up for, which I thought was great to see. It might sound silly, but I like to see my dogs think and then act, making their own careful choices without my input. Being in the position to be able to make sensible decisions takes time for some dogs, and I loved to see what came from that.

A special place to sit was at a gate to a field where there were usually Hereford cows, known for being gentle, slow and calm. Hagrid liked to sit by them and they'd quietly sniff each other. It was on this walk that Hagrid would have the opportunity to observe chickens as they wandered around a nearby farmyard. As well as a good number of chickens and cockerels, there were guinea fowl and ducks. It was noisy and this attracted Hagrid's attention.

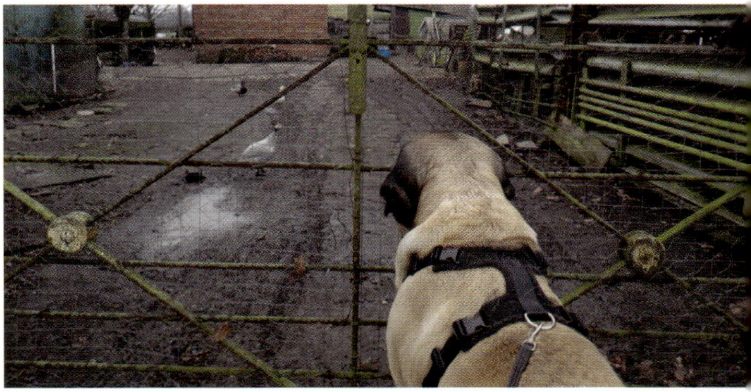

Hagrid watching fowl wander around and listening to the noises they made. Notice he's quite excited, standing tall and leaning forwards, with his ears up. Always observing him while he did this and taking note of his excitement levels on the day enabled me to know when to move on and when to stay. At times the fowl were further away and that made it easier for him to walk off.

We started out seeing the farm from a little way away down the track. But as the months passed, we began to extend the walk in different directions and have some other choices of where to go each time we came to the area. At first, we strolled past the farm on the other side of the road, giving Hagrid maximum space. We did this for the first few times, over months, and this was his first exposure to fowl. Within time the visits became more regular as he gained gradual exposure to the goings-on in the farmyard.

Hagrid needed a day at home now and then and, while it was important for him to get outside, it was up to me to find ways to make sure he could enjoy a *comfortable* walk. It was also great to listen when he didn't want to go out because there'd be reasons, even though it may not have been evident why at the time. On these days, we'd usually do something low-key and enriching at home to add interest to his life. Observing and making changes so a dog is able to enjoy both going out and staying home is worthwhile and fulfilling for them.

It was highly exciting for him, and he became vocal once or twice, so distracting him and moving on before he reached the over excitement stage was necessary. He learned from this and found that sitting and observing the fowl was enough, and later was even able to walk away of his own accord without my suggestion or intervention.

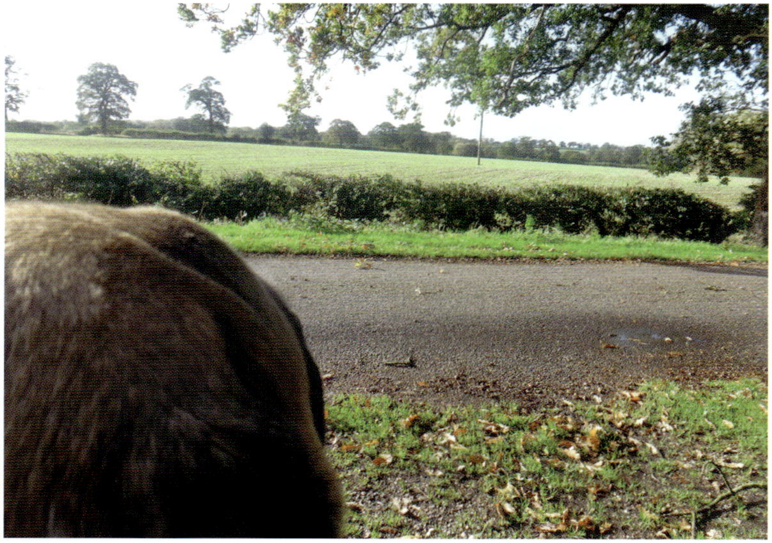

This was one of Hagrid's places to sit and observe. Just as humans sit down to take in the beauty of nature, I'm sure dogs appreciate things like this too.

Over time, Hagrid began to sit down even on the shortest of walks. Some days he'd sit because he lacked confidence or got stuck at certain places. That was okay though. I gently tried encouraging him to go a little further or take other routes around the same area. It's important to know the dog and find out reasons for sitting; some may feel pain and need to go back and sometimes that's what Hagrid needed.

Sitting down on walks was Hagrid's time. It was his walk and if he wanted to do that, that's what we did. After a while, typically five minutes or so, I'd say 'do you want to go?' And if he was ready to move on, we'd usually walk on a bit further and sit somewhere else. In some places he'd tell me if he didn't want to get up yet, also sometimes I needed him to go back! Then we'd move on at his pace; slowly. We enjoyed being together, being still and quiet. I'd squat down next to him and he'd rest his head on my shoulder. I miss those days, special moments and I genuinely miss Hagrid. I can still imagine this minute how every bit of him felt. The tears roll.

When we reached the van, Hagrid would sit again, adjusting to the fact the walk was over, which usually took a couple of minutes - not too long to wait - then he'd be ready to get in.

> Some dogs need time to adjust to the fact the walk is coming to an end and is over.

He'd stand in his large crate, waiting for a slow massage on his back and legs, so I'd massage as much of him as I could reach. He looked forward to this each time he got into the van after a walk. Once that was done he'd settle down on his bed.

Sitting on walks for other dogs

Dogs sit down because they need to and for whatever reason, it's part of their communication repertoire and a strong signal so it's worth listening to. They could be tired, in pain, overwhelmed, communicating with another dog, losing confidence, not wanting to go (there will be a reason), or simply because they want to stop, for example.

Hagrid taught me that sitting time was valuable for being calm and level, so I tried it with Pogo, because at the time she was a highly energetic and stressed dog. At first I could see these times, although for her they were fleeting moments, made a small but noticeable difference. She'd have a glimmer of calm, which began to grow. When Pogo became highly excited, I shortened her long lead, squatted down beside her and gently supported her until she seemed to slow her inner pace down, beginning to focus on where she was. She didn't always sit, and I didn't ask her to; she chose how she needed to be. Gradually, Pogo was able to settle for more extended periods and eventually sitting down became part of our walk just as it was with Hagrid. She even learned the need to stop and regulate herself, on the lead of course but wow, this was powerful. It's often a tool I use for dogs that need help in that way.

As time went by it wasn't always possible to sit where Pogo wanted. Indeed, it wasn't always possible to sit when Hagrid wanted to! But then as I knew my dogs, I knew when it was genuine and needed or for other reasons. At times, they sat just because they could, perhaps to delay ending our time out together, so in these moments I was empathetic and gently encouraged them to walk on with me. It made me smile how they were clever enough to use sitting to lengthen their walks but it wasn't an issue for either of us to move on. They could stop and take a few seconds, standing, sitting if they chose to but also resting. It can help a dog to be still and grounded if they're flighty. Please note – I call it 'sitting time' but the dog chooses what position they adopt within the short break. We manage well without commands.

I find the break is more than likely going to be momentary and happens only if my dog chooses. However, in time these breaks became a regular feature of a walk. If a dog was unable to stop at first, as with Pogo, just briefly pausing to tie my shoe, for example, could be enough to give her time to think a little and slow down. That way there was no focus on her. But it needed to be an honest and considered stop to make sense. Over months this was built upon. And while useful for some dogs, maybe it didn't need to be a part of every walk or for every dog. Dogs know when something is unnatural, and when we're acting, so taking a break needs to be valid to them. Having a valid reason or choosing the right moment seems viable to dogs, rather than just stopping in a barren environment. It's often easier for them if there is something to sniff and they don't feel exposed and vulnerable, as this encourages a natural break in the walk. See fall2016.iaabcjournal.org/train-sit-reconsider-relevance for more.

Scavenging

Some dogs will roll on, or near, a dead animal and/or urinate around the area. Hagrid found food and dead animals now and then, and sometimes I'd need to put a limit on the lead so he wasn't able to reach them. He respected this because he was able to have what he'd found at other times, or do what he needed to do. Care needs to be taken for dogs with allergies so this will depend on the individual. The times when Hagrid did find food or a dead animal were so rare that it didn't seem to make any difference to his overall health. His quality of life was what mattered most and being able to be a dog at times enriched his life.

Not everything was appropriate

Using my observational skills, if I were to see a discarded takeaway and didn't think it appropriate, in this situation I'd bring the long line in well before he could reach it, creating much more space between him and it, casually as we walked. I'd keep the boundary on the lead until he was ready to turn away and go in a different direction. And that's one of the benefits of occasionally letting dogs have some of the things that they find. They accept it far more easily when they can't have something. Like people, dogs will try harder to get hold of an item that's made into a forbidden fruit. It's a process of being reasonable and fair.

Throwing objects for dogs

Having a ball or object thrown for them usually excites a dog and it's often done for that reason; to keep them occupied, as well as for exercise. Excitement of any kind, whether positive or negative, creates the same physical and chemical reaction, it impacts on the body and mind. But this impact, which can show up many years later, is not always associated with what has gone on before.

Too much chasing, jumping, twisting, suddenly stopping, swift turns and other running around can result in a dog prematurely showing stiffness, injuries, muscle wasting, dragging his legs or other problems later in life. Problems can be both external and internal. For some dogs though, this becomes addictive and when something is thrown they have to chase because it's instinctive for them to pursue fast moving objects. A few can become so wound-up and focus just on what they're chasing to the exclusion of everything else. In turn, many people view exercise as fun, and do this in a way to keep a dog fit and active or as a form of control. Some see it as an easy way to tire a dog out. However, in the wild it's rare for any animal to chase for the sake of it, especially in a way to wear themselves out.

As a side note for some perspective; an interesting observational account of street dogs in India by Sindhoor Pangal shows what dogs do when people have minimal influence on their daily lives: www.livesofstreeties.com.

In the natural world, the frequency of coerced chasing where an object is thrown wouldn't happen. In creating sports for dogs, over the years, there is a cost to them, and us too. This cost affects us in numerous ways – emotionally and physically – and may also result in unnecessary vet bills to repair the damage caused.

Put simply, dogs don't need to chase objects or balls or participate in other fast sports that have been created for them, but it seems quite often people want to see them run, because we've become accustomed to it. By the age of ten, and sometimes before then, many dogs have stiff legs, arthritis and other physical ailments that are likely to result from over exertion.

According to Rialland, et. al (2012)[1], the prevalence of osteoarthritis (OA) in the U.S. canine population is concerning; nearly 20% of adult dogs, and 80% of dogs eight years or older have arthritis. There are several reasons why some might develop arthritis and other physical ailments: over-exercise is one of those. It can put an incredible load on the whole body internally as well as externally. For that reason, I am sensible with my dogs and find with moderate exercise and reducing stressors they are far less likely to have creaky joints at a relatively young age.

Some dogs might be more susceptible to certain illnesses than others due to their breed or genetics. Over-exercise, including chasing balls or other toys, tugging games, rough play and so on, can aggravate any existing conditions and might even cause their early onset. So it's possible that these illnesses could be avoided, and most certainly delayed, with the right care.

Stiffness and arthritis can at least be put off until much later or even prevented, by having a suitable balance between diet, exercise and lifestyle choices. Even if a dog has developed some illnesses, it's not too late to make a difference by adopting the practices shown in this book. It's something we did with Jaffa, who suffered from several illnesses that Cavaliers are prone to; Syringomyelia being one of these. Jaffa's symptoms almost disappeared thanks to changes we made in her lifestyle. These adjustments included observing her, taking note of her signals and language, making dietary changes, limiting stress in her life and watching for signs that she'd done enough, before becoming tired out. It's all too easy to push a dog too far due to our expectations of them.

I used to be a marathon runner and trained hard for several years. Exercise was an addiction for me and the reason I stopped was because of picking up several recurring injuries. This is my personal experience, and I've seen plenty of people and dogs who have similar issues when exercise has been unsuitable and/or too much. I listened to my body eventually, and now walk in moderation, rarely picking up injuries.

A note on addictions

What we know about addiction is that it's defined as a chronic brain disease, not natural, or what a dog would choose to do. If they are unable to have a walk without having a ball thrown, there's a problem.

Those who chase items too often, by which I mean more than three or so throws, or who run with other dogs on a regular basis for too long are more likely to

1. Rialland, P., Bichot, S., Moreau, M. et al. Clinical validity of outcome pain measures in naturally occurring canine osteoarthritis. BMC Vet Res 8, 162 (2012). https://doi.org/10.1186/1746-6148-8-162

have their prey drive heightened. This is often described as play, however, they, being essentially 'wired' will be less able to relax and sleep well.

Being weaned off addictive activities that create high arousal is possible. Allowing a dog to just carry a ball may help in the interim. Being rolled along the ground a couple of times could be acceptable for a few who are hooked on them. Some accept it straight away when an activity is stopped; it depends on their individual personality. Others may require a more structured programme to ensure they can be weaned off gradually, thereby avoiding unnecessary suffering. Please refer to the contacts at the back of this book if help is needed with any of this.

At first, I was concerned that my dogs may become bored with having less exercise, around half an hour a day depending on the dog at that point in time, their age, health and other factors. I was pleasantly surprised, however, to find they are much more settled and able to sleep more than most of my dogs in the past who had had much more high intensity, long duration exercise and lots going on in their daily lives. I have found that accepting and adjusting to this, observing and learning about them has helped them to live happier lives in the long run.

> When ball throwing/chasing is regular and goes on for too long (more than a few throws) it can become addictive. Just as we are not born with cigarettes in our mouths, neither are dogs born with balls in theirs.

A dog being engaged with sniffing in an environment he finds enriching offers far more appropriate stimulation than anything we can give them. As long as it's interesting and they can take their time, being inquisitive is self-satisfying. Throwing balls for dogs and encouraging them to chase is something that's been around for many years. Some have been taught to play with a ball rather than learning how to deal with life, often at cost to the dog's health.

Just as I experienced when constantly chasing various stimulants or highs, a dog that does the same is less able to switch off and rest as much as they need. They are likely to learn to react quickly, sometimes without thinking, and chase other moving things we'd prefer them not to go after. Keeping a dog highly active will encourage this behaviour. I, like many people, would prefer it if my dogs don't chase cats, farm animals and the like, so steer away from toys that create excitement. Dogs simply don't need high arousal.

Final thoughts

Building from a place of pleasure, happiness and contentment on walks, dogs can develop an interest in life. At first, this could lead to fearfulness, which is what happened with Hagrid, because he suddenly saw the world through fresh eyes. He required some extra support and gentle limits at this time. Dogs need time to observe what is happening at a distance, and this can promote confidence. To merely observe at a suitable distance, one that is usually much further away than we might imagine a dog requires, is a necessary treat for most of them.

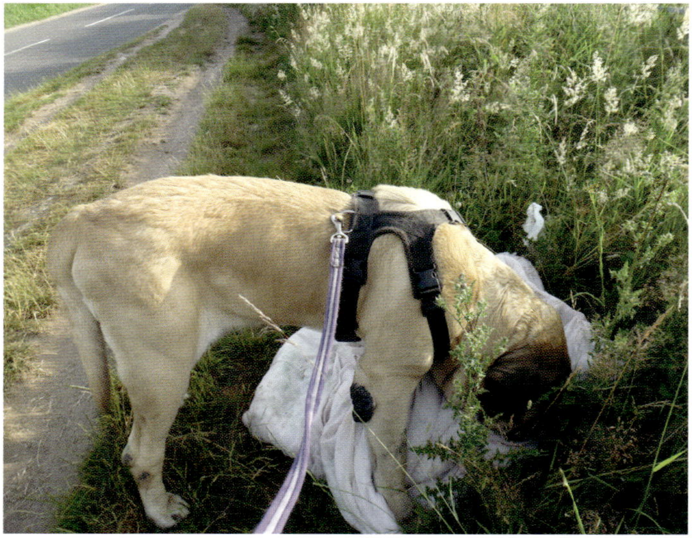

An item Hagrid found and chose to investigate. He became deeply engrossed in sniffing a quilt that had been left at the side of the road! Here the boundary is the lead, so he is safe near the road.

Hagrid, like a lot of dogs, had been told what, how and what not to do, but now he was given a chance to work things out for himself, so there was a period of him not knowing how to respond. At this time he was supported, with limited choices so he wasn't overwhelmed. I found that some unwanted behaviours arose from this newfound liberty as a result of him being scared because at first he didn't always know the best way to respond. The sudden change made it scary for me too.

When this happens there's a tendency for controlling them. Being empathetic, open and available, at the same time going slowly, helped Hagrid and I to feel safe and able to trust during this time.

Interestingly, limits can facilitate greater freedom. When children have safe limits, they are free to express themselves and play within a secure environment. Without boundaries, a child lacks safety and will be less inclined to engage in open, creative play. Likewise, reasonable limitations allow a dog to experience freedom safely and can be expanded as the dog settles. They can also be flexible and help a dog to return to safety, before expanding the perimeters again.

Sometimes this is needed so real progress can be made.

Key points

- There is a significant difference between what is of interest to a dog and what is of interest to a human.
- Walks are a chance for individual time with my dogs; we can be together, connected and in-tune.
- Being taught to use a long line effectively in a nurturing, sensitive and compassionate way makes so much difference to the way a dog behaves.
- We found quiet places to go with Hagrid at first, because going for a walk was enough in itself without the distractions of people, dogs, traffic and other animals.
- All kinds of places can hold interest for a dog, if they're allowed to explore.
- From a long distance he could watch for a little time, without reacting.
- Being in the position to be able to make sensible choices takes time for some dogs.
- Sometimes I felt embarrassed at the time we stood there while he watched. It seemed like a long time, but doing that a few times helped Hagrid build a positive, unobtrusive picture of humans.
- Training myself to respond calmly to situations really benefitted Hagrid.
- Challenging situations do arise, that's part of life. It's what we do or don't do that counts.
- Hagrid's barking was an advance on his slithering along the ground behaviour.
- He didn't bark at people who carried on with whatever they were doing, rather than giving us attention.
- Hagrid didn't like being barked at and would want to go home straight away if it happened. No dog likes having to bark or being barked at.
- It's all too easy to push a dog too far due to our expectations of them.

Key points (continued)

- Space and a relaxed approach can do wonders for our ability to think, assess and make better choices.
- Dogs can have very different needs and walking them separately is a great way to meet these.
- Walking away and leaving dogs to deal with a situation is going to make them less confident and worry more on walks.
- Fear can suppress communication.
- Like people, dogs will try harder to get hold of something if it's made into a forbidden fruit. It's a process of being reasonable and fair.
- Excitement of any kind, whether positive or negative, creates a physical and chemical reaction that impacts the body and mind.
- Having time living as individuals in their own right is healthy and gives dogs a chance to develop self-assurance.
- In the natural world, the frequency of coerced chasing where an object is thrown wouldn't happen.
- Being engaged with sniffing in an environment he finds enriching offers far more appropriate stimulation for a dog than anything we can give them.
- Walking dogs individually means that it's possible to observe, get to know their preferences and notice changes as the walk progresses.
- When they come too close to other dogs, it can be harder to express their feelings adequately and be acknowledged.
- Dogs sit down because they need to for whatever reason. It's part of their repertoire and a strong signal so it's worth listening to.
- Limits can facilitate greater freedom. When children have safe limits, they are free to express themselves and play, within a secure environment.

Chapter 8

Hagrid's cake and cat walk

This story is a practical example of how understanding Hagrid helped him on a typical walk. On this particular route, we walked down a quiet overgrown alley; not an ideal place to meet anyone but it was a risk I sometimes chose to take as we rarely saw anyone, providing I was careful with the timing. Occasionally we'd see people, and I'd make sure there was sufficient space for Hagrid, so he didn't become flustered and worry, lose his confidence and want to go home.

Seeing people just once in a while helped him build his self-confidence, trusting in the fact that no one would invade his space and knowing he had a choice whether to meet them or not. When someone did speak to us in passing or stopped for a brief chat, he was in a much better position to deal with it and often chose to distance himself from them, although not always.

There was still some underlying apprehension in Hagrid, so I learnt how to offend people least when asking them to give us space. There were certain people I knew I was able to trust to be around him and some even understood enough to allow him to sniff them while resisting the temptation to touch or stare at him. This helped him gain confidence. Getting it right most of the time goes a long way to help with those odd times when someone may take you by surprise. Often, I've found that a dog deals with the one-off time when someone doesn't respond to our requests to leave the dog alone.

Because of Hagrid's issues, it sometimes took him a few seconds to notice (through sense of smell) if anyone was in the vicinity, so that also helped with management. Still, I didn't like to put this pressure on him; hence going out at quiet times of the day or in less pleasant weather conditions. Imagine how unsettling it must feel knowing someone has gone past and you noticed too late. He occasionally seemed suspicious, strangely when nothing was happening, and I guess it could well be due to times he'd realised (again through sense of smell) that people or dogs had passed him by after the event. What a confusing world he must have inhabited.

Down the alleyway, I guided him through the zigzagged railings by careful use of the lead. As my granddaughter often said, "you're his guide person". Hagrid relied heavily on his nose to gather information about his surroundings. Although his eyes worked to some extent, he didn't seem to process visual stimuli very well for some reason.

On this particular occasion Hagrid's nose led him to quite a sizeable half-eaten cupcake, which he soon devoured, and I waited while he had a good rummage around, making sure every crumb had gone. After a few minutes, he walked on a metre or so before backtracking. I do mean minutes – he was slower than your average Mastiff – at least the ones I've met. So having gone back, he enthusiastically began to sniff the fence with great concentration. I noticed a cat peering over a wall opposite to where Hagrid was sniffing. What a picture it made. The cat was observing intently as he tried desperately to locate the scent it was giving off. He sensed it was fresh cat. When Hagrid was so absorbed in this way, it gave me information that something had been there recently or was perhaps still nearby. After a minute, he suddenly got a whiff of the cat and noticed it on top of the wall, which fortunately was some height above him. He became even more animated, keen to get closer to the cat. As soon as he attempted to climb the wall, the cat thought better of watching and vanished from sight.

Okay, so now I thought we were off again, having already spent at least five minutes in this short alley but… just hang on said Hagrid, I need to go back to see if anyone has thrown down more cupcakes. So back a few feet we went. Sniff, sniff, snuffle, snuffle. Hmm, no more cupcakes. Maybe more cats then.

After another five minutes of checking out where he'd found it, he decided that he had finished with cats, but then needed a rest. He sat down, and his nose began gently twitching – utterly different sniffing from before. The sniffing seemed to be mild interest in the general environment and, after yet more minutes, we moved toward the end of the alley where I spied the cupcake wrapper in thick ivy growing alongside the wall. I wondered what would happen.

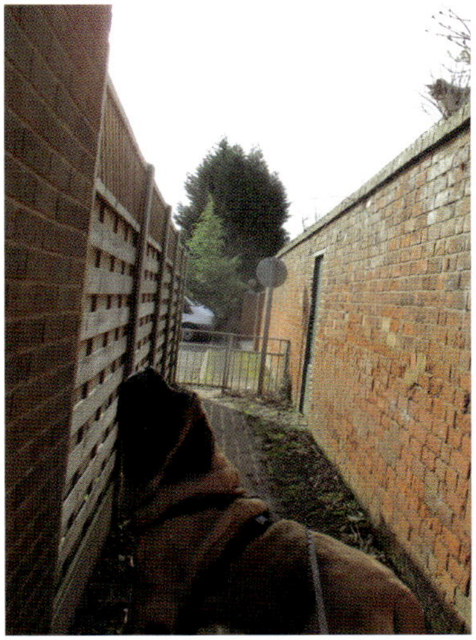

"I can smell cat."

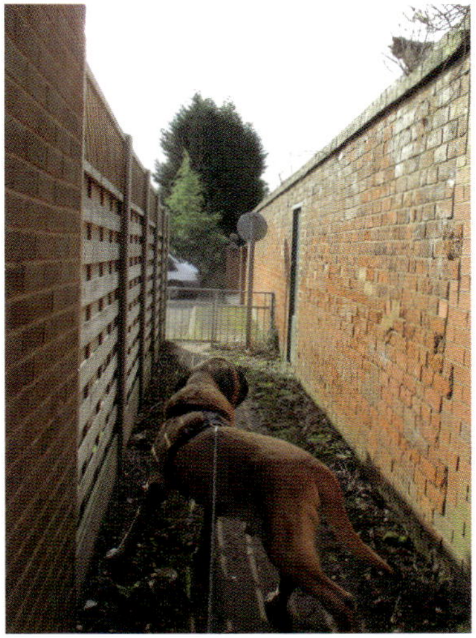

"There's the cat!"

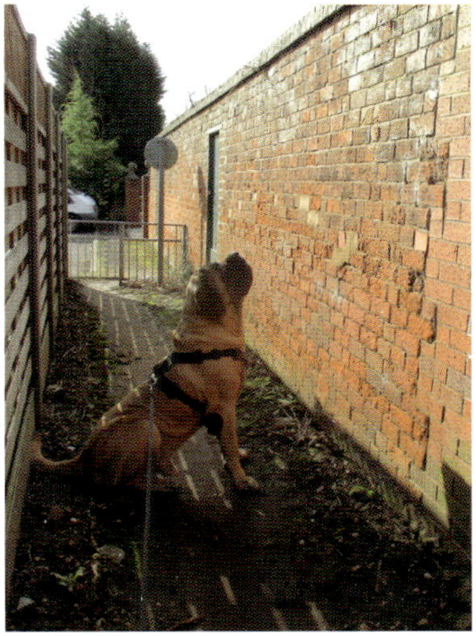

"Where's it gone?"

Showing how long the alleyway is and Hagrid snuffling around in search of the cake wrapper.

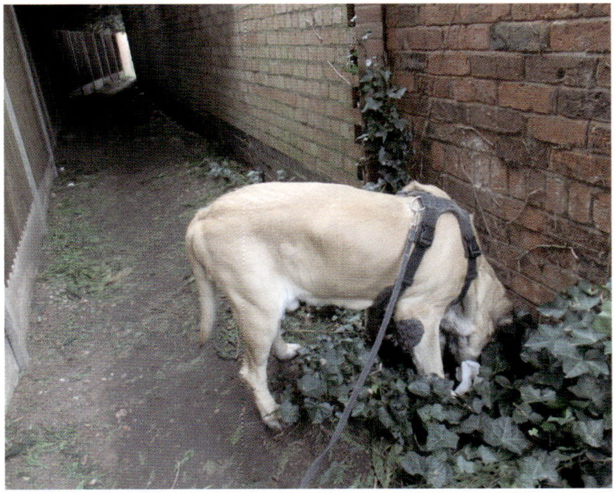

Length of alley.

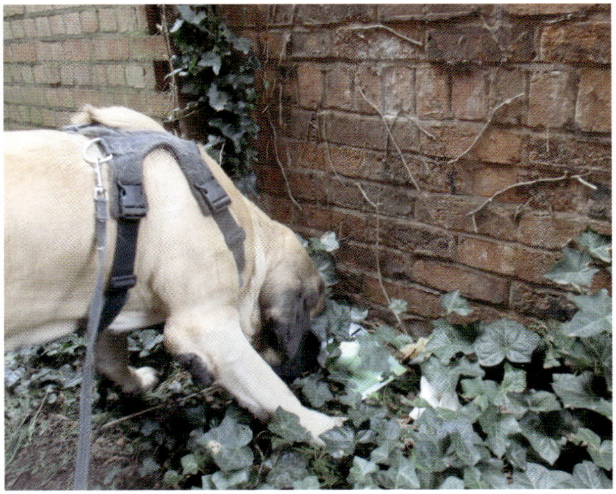

Finding the cupcake wrapper.

Soon (that's Hagrid soon!) after he'd caught a whiff of something good he began mooching in the ivy and was slowly working his way down to the discarded wrapper. And then 'Bingo!' his big head landed alongside the wrapper, then on top of it. GONE.

When I saw the wrapper, it only seemed fair to allow Hagrid to have it because he was using so much thought and energy to problem solve. I could have put a boundary on the lead to prevent him getting it, but why? Having used limits on the lead regularly, Hagrid responded well to them and respected the communication between us. On our walks I had an advantage over him and could see ahead, so stayed vigilant and if I saw him sniffing intently, it was usually possible to spot the item of interest before he had the chance to track it down, but did my best not to spoil his enthusiasm.

Because I know each of my dogs, I can use my judgment regarding what is likely to do them harm and allow them occasionally to have bits of food and other things dogs find tasty when we are out. If I had regularly and unreasonably restricted Hagrid's access to things he was drawn to he'd probably become frustrated and if Hagrid was attracted to something, he could easily use his strength and weight (thirteen stone of it!) to get it and bolt it down before I stopped him. The kind of 'give and take' scenario I've just explained works so well. If we allow dogs a little freedom, supporting their decisions and engaging with them, they are more likely to feel good about themselves. This, in turn, enables confidence-building, respect for our wishes and enhances the relationship.

During the time Hagrid had his head in the ivy taking in various smells and then devouring the wrapper, a lady walked past us. As I'd been involved and focused on what Hagrid was doing I didn't speak to her, but when he'd finished his wrapper, a few seconds later he'd picked up on her scent. However, he barely noticed her probably because his recent activity was still being processed and took priority. He sat down again for a short time, just being there and registering his environment by air scenting before we headed back home. We were out for hardly half an hour, but for Hagrid, it was a high-quality walk.

The point of this story is to show how enriching and fulfilling a short, slow walk can be for a dog and carer too (sad I know!). And for what the dog gets from a simple activity, which at one time I may not have registered. Instead, I would have been focused on the energy spent for my dog.

This walk had such quality; he was using his brain, his skills and that's everything. Okay, so Hagrid wasn't your average run-of-the-mill dog, but it's the little things that generally go unnoticed or can be taken for granted and those things hold a lot of meaning for a dog. Taking time to slowly let Hagrid explore, backtracking when he wanted to, was another way of giving him a choice about 'his' walk.

The key message here is that if we give opportunities and choices to dogs within reasonable limits, then they are more likely to make their own sensible decisions and come away from scenarios and items when we really need them to. It's important to reiterate that we need to assess the environment and guide our dogs away from unsuitable finds, preferably ahead of time, but if we give in to them now and then, they end up respecting our decisions when they are needed. Of course, it's paramount that our animals don't end up seriously ill or worse, because they've eaten poison or something that is toxic to them, so please remain vigilant.

In summary, I think it's fair to say that walks were alive for Hagrid and me, and a big part of what we did. It really can be like that for others if they can see the potential creativity in it.

CHAPTER 9

Choices

Helping a dog to develop awareness and independence is amazing. Observing the changes as he graduates from being told when and how to do things into making his own simple choices is so rewarding. Making decisions might not always be easy at first, especially when much of the dog's life may have been quite controlled up until this point, but a dog that's allowed to carry out natural behaviour without fear of being told off or over-controlled, will start to show happiness in subtle ways. Always having choices can be stressful, so gently does it, especially when a dog is in transition from having few.

Simple decisions could be choosing when to go out, where to go for a walk (within reason), and when and where to go to the toilet. Around the house, a dog could be allowed to decide where to lie down, when to go out and come in, and when and where to eat. When boundaries are applied to these choices, it could then be, for example, the choice of where to sleep, limited to one or two rooms. It's easy to close a door or dog gate; provided they are used to this, that's a boundary dogs can understand without the need for us to say much.

Throughout, a dog still requires limits that will vary depending on where he is with his experience and skill to deal effectively with what he meets. Putting in place some physical boundaries promotes understanding and still allows a dog to have freedom, within those limits.

It's worth restating that at first, this could lead to fearfulness because now he suddenly sees the world through fresh eyes. For Hagrid, going slowly gave him time to see what was happening, at a distance. When a dog is given a chance to work it out for himself, there will probably be a period of not knowing what to do or how. Some unwanted behaviours may result from this new found freedom and can scare us humans because we don't always know the best way to respond. But the dog is scared too. This situation can create a tendency for us to over-control because we are scared. Being empathetic, open and available will help him to feel safe and able to trust.

Giving total freedom could be as confusing as being given strict controls.

As mentioned before, limits can actually give more freedom. When we put in safe limits for children they're free to express themselves and play more freely because they are safe, and there isn't that worry or risk of danger. A child without boundaries lacks security and will be less inclined to engage in open, creative play because it creates insecurity. Likewise, boundaries allow a dog to experience freedom safely. Limiting things at the start helps a dog to return to safety, creating a solid base to expand upon after. Sometimes this is needed before real progress can be made. As we observe their changes in behaviour, we can decide how to deal with it sympathetically. It's a gradual, two-way, process for both dog and carer.

A dog that's been controlled may seem well behaved. He will do as he is told, but if he's asked to sit and is uncomfortable with his surroundings, he may become agitated, and try to get up, remove himself from the situation, fidget, pant or jump up only to be told to sit again. Over time, the dog may give up trying to communicate what he really wants to do. This is often considered as obedient but really the dog is repressing his natural urge to respond to the situation. They are always giving us these messages about how they're feeling. Replacing fixed commands with empathy, understanding and flexible boundaries can lead to a remarkable improvement in a dog's behaviour. Accepting the dog for all his behaviours and allowing outlets within safe limits will lead to a freer way of living together. A chance for us to gain insight into how they really feel.

When out on walks, a long line can give a dog great support if used sensitively. There are many times when dogs need our input in our world.

By gently guiding them in the intended direction, through lead handling skills, use of positioning and body language, indicating where to go and waiting

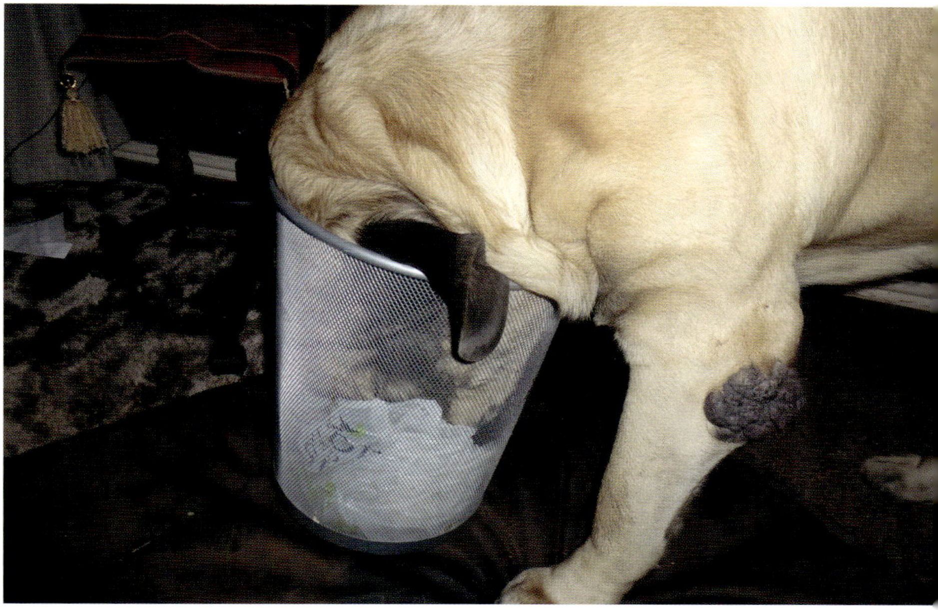

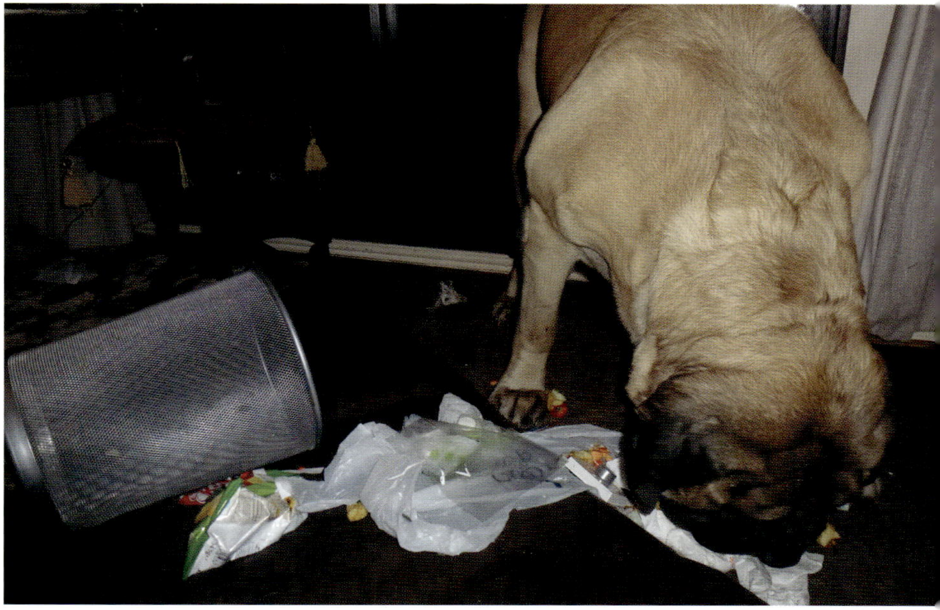

An example of choices in the house: investigating the bin. On this occasion I'd collected the bins ready to be emptied when something caught Hagrid's attention. It was fine for me to clear up after he'd finished and he wasn't a dog who usually chose to go into the bins. If I didn't want him to make these kinds of choices then it was my responsibility to stop it being possible in the first place by keeping the bin out of his way, or step in before this happened.

for them to respond, they have the chance and time to think for themselves. Sometimes the dog can make the choices, other times the handler can, or will need to.

Each dog is an individual and will progress at their own pace. A dog, given choices when they previously haven't been, is likely to show some happiness in different ways. For example, having a little bounce of mild excitement when on a walk, cocking his leg when he hadn't before, turning around to look at the handler, or scratching the ground with his back legs after having a wee. A dog may hold himself more upright and confident, walk tall or have a relaxed posture. These are all subtle behaviours that may emerge.

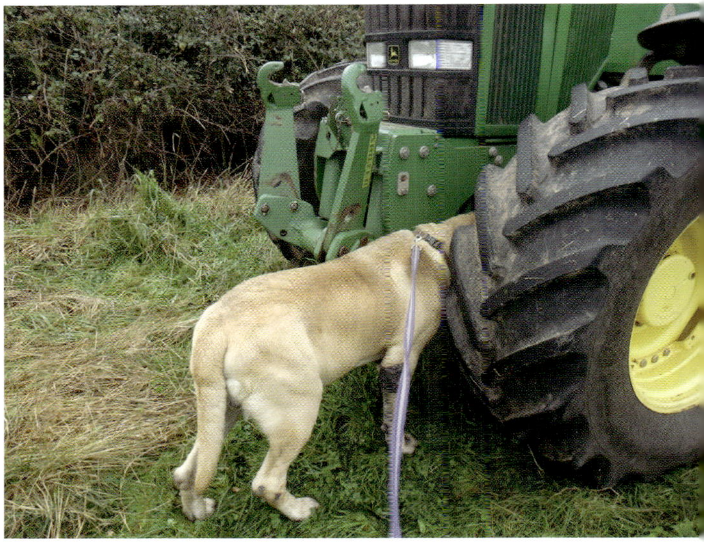

The farmer had parked his tractor in a field that we walked in, and it came with fresh and interesting smells in which Hagrid was very interested. Often this kind of thing added so much to his walks.

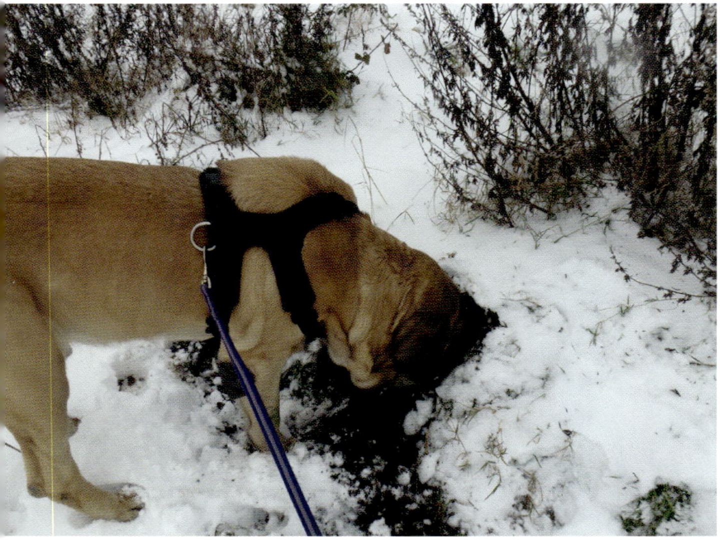

Hagrid thoroughly engaged in smells in the snow, digging down to find out more, carrying out his natural behaviours.

Chapter 10

Water

Water is great fun for most dogs, it is cooling and refreshing, plus it's great to see them wading in. This was Hagrid's 'thing'.

Like many dogs, Hagrid loved the water and it had the potential to excite him, therefore I needed to be mindful when he was in the water. This is because, like many dogs, he could get carried away in the excitement and become obsessed by it. Being aware of this gave me a chance to think ahead and be prepared.

Shortly after Hagrid came to live with us, we went on a walk by a river. He watched, both perplexed and focused. It was evident he had never seen anything like this before, which his previous owners later confirmed. The simple movement of the water intrigued him. While we were linked together by the long line, he walked into the river at a shallow point and after a while became fixated on his front legs as the water swirled around them. I wonder how it felt for him; the water's energy, its power and the sensations made on its journey down the river. Water was exciting for Hagrid, so I needed to pay attention: he was rather insistent that we should get there whenever he smelt any in the vicinity, and I could get pulled in!

One time, quite early on, we were near the river when Hagrid (who was still on-lead) took me by surprise and suddenly jumped in. He was out of his depth, which took him by surprise. Being so excited about water had taken him out of his 'thinking brain'. He began to sink and panicked, climbing up a steep bank to get out. It took a joint effort to hoist him up onto dry land, and I learned that he was not an efficient swimmer.

Seeing bubbles floating by had taken Hagrid to another level emotionally, which he hadn't experienced before, so he wasn't familiar with the concept of water and how it behaved. Because Hagrid panicked when out of his depth and climbed up where he did, he must have strained a front leg and, for a whole week afterwards, limped. If thinking rationally, he'd probably have noticed a nearby bank that was much lower.

In time, when Hagrid was calm, he was in a position to make rational decisions.

We learned that his front right leg was weak due to a previous operation, but this injury was a result of being over stimulated and was a case of overconfidence coupled with little experience. When a dog is thinking clearly, he can make sensible choices. These times of being overwhelmed are worth noting in terms of the dog learning and coping. Keeping calm and helping them resist temptation to become over-excited gives the dog the opportunity to make appropriate decisions and this was the aim in Hagrid's case.

In the beginning whenever visiting water, after a short while he would become a little over-excited caught up in the energy he was experiencing. I would call him over and after a few seconds he'd reluctantly come out, move away from the water and into the woods where he calmed down enough to sniff and explore. Several minutes later we'd return and he'd go back in. This second time he was more relaxed about the water.

From times like these, I learned the importance of timing: how to read Hagrid more closely, to observe him, ask him to come out before he got over-excited and unable to respond. This meant shorter times in and near the water. He learned, in time, to come out of his own accord before becoming overwhelmed.

That was a huge leap forward, to be able to self-regulate like that. We could go exploring together and on walks to a local river at a shallow spot, where both of us could feel safe.

After Hagrid had a taste for being in water, it seemed like he could almost sense when he was near it! Each time he became aware of water, even at a distance, he was very determined to get there. Unclipping Hagrid's lead was never an option because of his lack of awareness, which had been down to his health problems. It wasn't always appropriate to go to the water's edge; we needed more distance so that he wasn't tempted to pull me in.

This resulted in a lessening of his enthusiasm gradually, over the months. Hagrid accepted that sometimes we went right to a water source where he could go in, as long as he wasn't intently dragging me. Usually, although we were in the vicinity, we didn't go close enough for paddling, and he accepted this after a while.

We made the most of opportunities like floodwater. Hagrid could spend many happy times in flooded fields or in big puddles after heavy rain, which was safe and helped him a lot. Water was in unexpected places and we could enjoy it for a little before moving on.

Just as we'd worked gradually with introductions to people, we took the time to do the same with water. Sometimes we went to a place where there was a nearby river or a pond, but not so close for Hagrid to insist that we went in. All the time I'd watch Hagrid's levels of excitement because they were my guide to how he was reacting and keeping in control. Before he reached the stage of being unable to regulate his emotions, we'd move further away.

Hagrid's tail was a real giveaway sign to his level of arousal and would curl up into a C shape when he was most excited. Other signs were his ears standing up and moving closer together. He'd also become more intent, which I could feel immediately through the lead.

That's why I like my dogs to express how they're feeling. I can gauge the intensity of how they react to a situation then handle them the best way for their emotional well-being. If I taught them not to react by controlling them, then I wouldn't see their movements to understand how they were feeling. I'd be suppressing those feelings, their natural urge to move, which could either lead to them finding other outlets for their frustration or becoming ill over time.

I found that if I allowed him to have a little of what he wanted, such as have a dip in the river, rather than completely cutting him off, he was quicker to accept boundaries. This same principle applied to getting to know other animals, and to food Hagrid found while out on a walk. As a result, he'd be able to take himself away without a fuss, providing I'd given him enough time to satisfy his need. 'Enough' in this instance meant not getting in too deep or for too long, and so getting over-excited.

This learning comes over time and is a result of knowing a dog, having experiences with them, being patient and observing their communication.

Putting in boundaries

There were certain times when we needed to avoid water because Hagrid's skin condition had flared up. I felt for Hagrid when it wasn't possible for him to paddle in hot weather because going to the river was a fun part of his walk. In general, Mastiffs and some other big dogs don't always tolerate heat well. Going in water made a significant difference to Hagrid and I loved seeing how he'd spring back to life with the coolness of water!

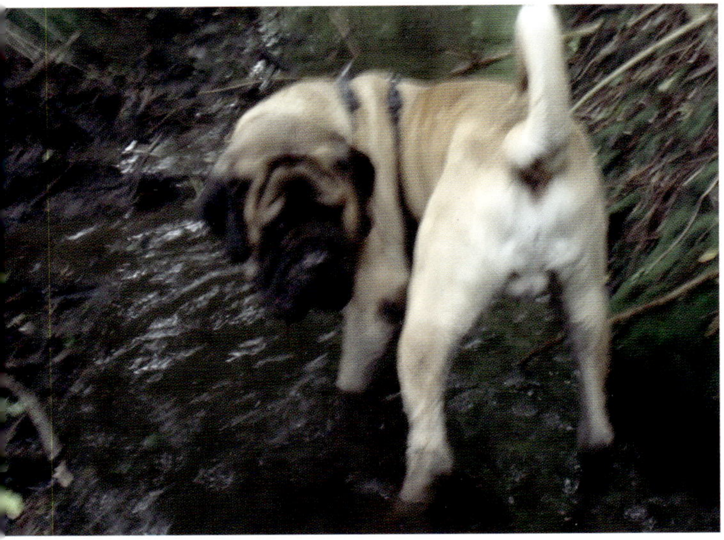

Although the photo is blurred it's easy to see that Hagrid was bemused by the sensations around his legs. Note his curled tail and the tension in his face and body compared to later photos where his body is much more relaxed being in water. This was one of the first times Hagrid had encountered water in this way.

A couple of months after Hagrid's leg operation, he wanted to go into the water while we were out on a walk. I used the lead to give him a boundary so he was able to go as far as three-quarters of the way up his legs. He accepted this, and that's what happens when given choices with fair boundaries.

Having occasional times of mild frustration (meaning frustration that doesn't go on for too long and cause real distress) is necessary for the development of any kind of compromise like this.

When Hagrid began to take me towards water, I often put a gentle stop in place on the lead especially on days he was very excited. He was frustrated at first, but when we walked at an appropriate distance from the water so he wasn't able to see it, there would be enough interest in the surrounding area to give him a different focus.

Swimming

Hagrid loved water, as you may have realised!

However, at one point he was limping, which was impacting his quality of life. This meant that he wasn't able to get out and about, so we tried to see if we could find a place where he could swim voluntarily in the hope that this would help him.

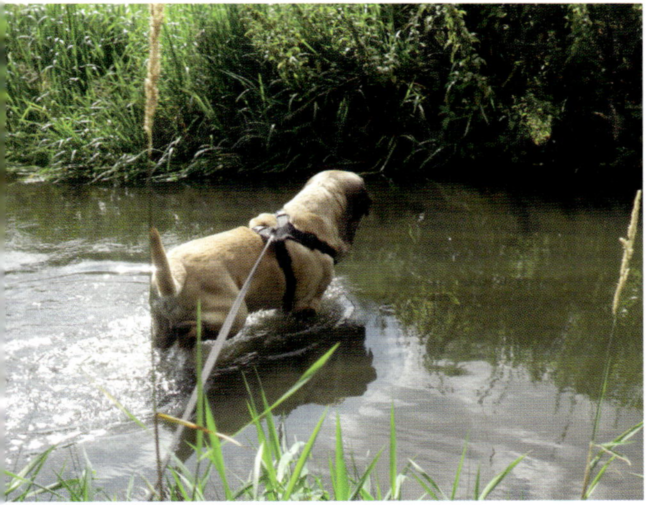

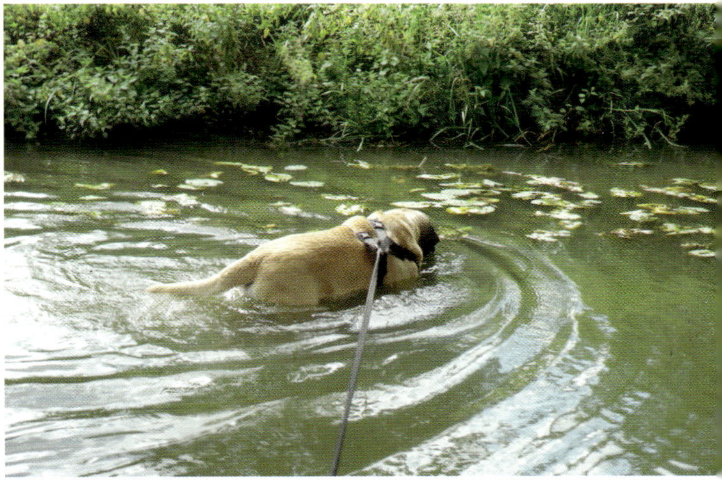

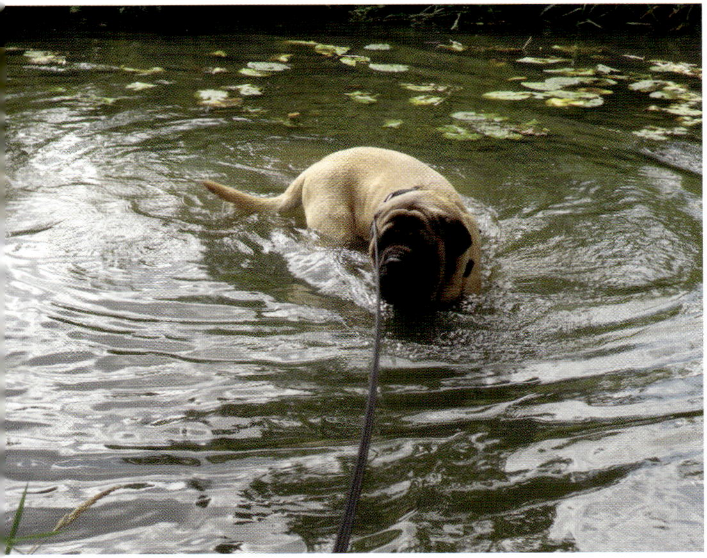

Hagrid's tail was high, which told me that he was quite excited by the water, so putting a boundary on the lead and waiting for him to respond was the best thing to do. It's possible to see when the boundary was applied in these photos. He got the message in his own time and turned around to come back out.

Kaos, another of my dogs, had been to canine hydrotherapy after she'd had a cruciate ligament operation. Sadly this had interrupted our relationship because I had to coerce her to go through an activity with which we were both uncomfortable. I was careful to bear this in mind for Hagrid and to do things differently.

Swimming or hydrotherapy is often advised for dogs after surgery, to help them recover. In the case of Kaos, I went along with it, but there were always questions for me about whether it suited her. Kaos didn't like it, and I wondered if her leg would heal if I didn't force her to go swimming, but was worried it would not heal properly. She was tense because she didn't want to get in – although that may have been different if she'd been given a choice and the time to get in and swim or not.

We went along to the sessions, week after week and Kaos was forced in, then coerced to stay and swim with someone she didn't know well. Not only did she hate going, but I hated taking her too. She did not choose to go in of her own accord, and eventually, I put a stop to it, essentially because she made it clear with her communication and I responded.

When the time came for Kaos to have the other cruciate ligament operated on, she recovered far more efficiently – without swimming – and was happier too. So was I. Being more relaxed benefitted her recovery. It's important to weigh up the pros and cons of each situation for all dogs, as they are so different. Our approach after this operation was to focus on stress reduction, care, regular and gentle massage, and stretching exercises that I did for her. We also introduced a gradual build up for her walks. This way of doing things was far more successful and came without the stress she'd endured the first time.

Hagrid not only trusted me, but he relied on me. He was a different dog to Kaos, and by now I'd learnt to observe my dogs' communication and listen to them. I was well aware of what to do if he decided he didn't like it at any point.

We found a place where horses swam, an indoor pool where they can be assisted by a weight-bearing harness, and asked about Hagrid swimming there. It all seemed relaxed, and when I asked about Hagrid's needs, everything was agreed. When we came to putting a buoyancy harness on him, that's where things started to change. There wasn't one large enough, so we made one out of two of them, which was the best we could do given what was available.

With hindsight, waiting around while we tried on harnesses was all we should have put him through that day. Instead, he was put into the water to swim. He was attached to a rope, one person either side of him, and was encouraged and pulled into the water. Once in, he tried to scramble up the sides to get out.

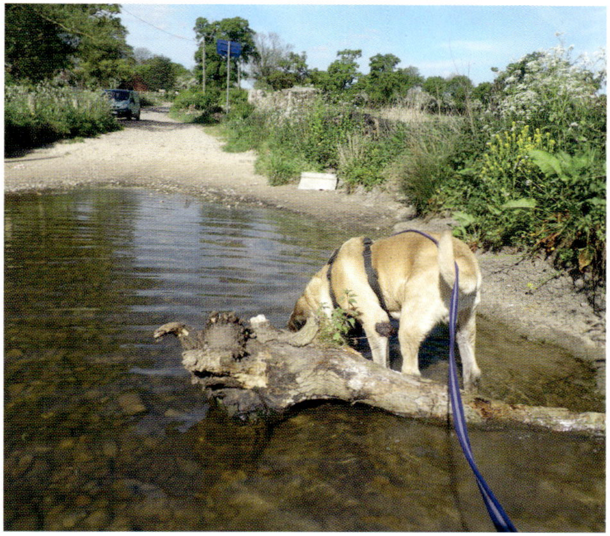

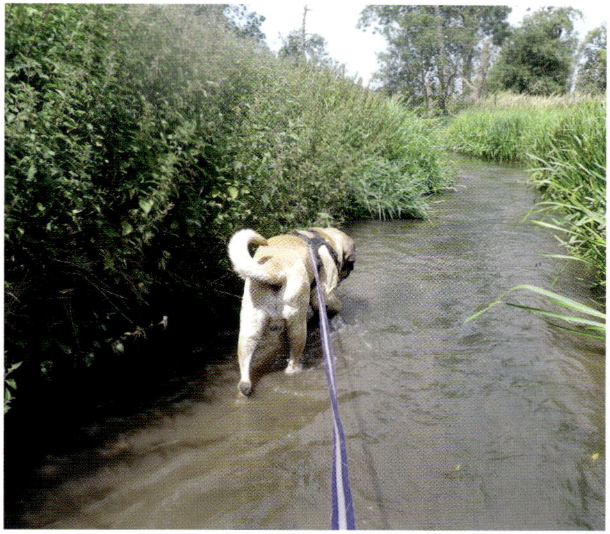

Hagrid enjoying exploring a local ford. He had options and a choice of routes to take and I'd go in with him.

He was just overwhelmed and didn't want to do it. Several others shouted encouragement to Hagrid from the sides of the pool. Sadly, it was an awful experience for him, and for me too.

Why hadn't I said stop? I had frozen in disbelief and couldn't find my voice.

I was there to help him but I certainly didn't feel as though I was helping. He didn't want to leave me and go into the pool. He was uncertain, but I'm sure he'd have been okay if I'd gone in with him. I wished I had. From what others could see, things looked to be going well, but they didn't know it was wrong to force or coerce animals to do things, whereas I did.

It's not easy to stand up for yourself. It can be challenging, especially when the majority of people around you have different ideas and beliefs. That's been my experience, and something I really struggle with. I'd outlined at the start what I wanted and that I wasn't going to force Hagrid into the water, but I backed down when several people I didn't know were involved and I felt overpowered.

The one person that Hagrid believed in had led him into something unknown and scary; something he wasn't ready for. I know if I'd been on my own with no one around, we wouldn't have gone through with it. We didn't go back because it had been a negative experience, and this reminded me that swimming wasn't necessary, even for a dog that loves water. There were other ways, and a few weeks later we tried acupuncture as a support for the other things we'd set in place.

We all find some things difficult and this is another lesson Hagrid taught me. It has helped me to step back, look at what is going on and what I need to work on to keep those boundaries in place when it's tough. By being receptive to it, dogs can offer the same lessons too. I've learned to ask for time to think, and am still learning how to stand my ground and walk away if necessary – a work in progress, just like many life lessons can be. It's usually possible to come back later, and opportunities for a U-turn are not always available once the damage is done. Trusting my intuition is what I do now.

Swimming can be good for dogs, provided it's done on their terms, at their pace, and their communication is always respected.

CHAPTER 11

Tracking and exploring

I regularly think back to the fun and enjoyment Hagrid and I had and the incredible journey we shared. Tracking was a great part of our time together. Tracking is hiding an object with a scent and leaving a trail for the dog to follow. It can be enriching, while also building a connection with a dog in a way that's natural to them.

Hagrid seemed to really enjoy tracking and I allowed time and space for this part of his life. He would have a good time searching for the different items I'd planted for him. Hagrid liked being in our van and would wait in there happily while I made a trail. I'd be sure to walk back a different way so as not to cross the path I'd just taken and make the scent confusing. Then I'd open the doors and, with Hagrid safely on his long line, he'd be off; head down, hardly giving me a chance to close the van door.

This was Hagrid living in the fast lane! He walked fast for a few paces before slowing down to an even pace. Each time we did tracking together it was pleasantly exciting for him. He seemed to enjoy these little challenges, just as I did. I was always mindful not to over-excite him to the point that he became stressed or tired.

It's a delicate balance; some stimulation to help with enjoyment and quality of life, but not too much for a dog to become obsessive or exhausted. Less really is more. There wasn't a need to use exciting words, cues or to add emotion to our voices, it only put my dogs off. Tracking itself was the reward. We were in the moment with them and watched how they worked things out. There was no need for excessive praise; a low-key acknowledgment was enough.

Just a tiny bit of help was needed sometimes, and in a subtle way. It was interesting to watch him catch the smells and where they took him. He was great at tracking my scent. For many dogs it's possible to use another person's scent from your own, but Hagrid found it hard to trust people, so this wasn't for him. Dogs like Hagrid who have negative past experiences can struggle tracking a person with whom they don't feel safe. These are things learnt when tracking.

On one occasion, my son David was accompanying us on walks. We decided that David could lay a track, with himself at the end. Hagrid successfully tracked him and to witness his skill was fascinating. He approached the challenge by completing a large arc, approaching David from behind and advancing with uncertainty. I sensed that this was uncomfortable for both David and Hagrid so we decided not to do it again. Although nothing bad had happened, it looked to me as though Hagrid was worried about finding David, and David had found it quite uncomfortable as well. I respected and appreciated both of their needs.

One of the alternatives I found was to begin the day by walking Jaffa first. I'd take some of Hagrid's toys with me and put them down in places just off the track. At first I made the toys easy to find so that he could begin to work out what to do. Often, we can make activities like this a little too complicated and challenging for dogs, and in my experience it pays to start slowly and allow them to learn at a gentle pace, to aim for success.

A dog needs to feel satisfied to be able to build confidence. Roughly three short tracks, where they can see it being laid, was enough for most of my dogs in one session to start with. Much later, one longer path might be sufficient depending on the dog, but was always guided by their communication and body language.

This is a confidence-building activity for a dog, so if things are set up at the right level, then they can grow. It's possible to get carried away when seeing them doing well and set sights too high, so it's better to build up slowly and keep it simple. Going back to basics means they can be successful and have enjoyment.

I mention this because it can be pretty competitive when it comes to people and their dogs, for many reasons. Just as some have experienced pressure from their parents to succeed, or have wanted to drive children to do well, the same can happen with dogs.

Think about it; our world is driven by the desire to get the best results, the best life. It runs deep in our blood. But dogs don't care about any of this.

Looking closely in the top left of this picture, it's possible to see the object Hagrid's tracking. When he found it, he picked this up and carried it home. There was no great excitement from either of us once he found it. Instead, he showed his pleasure how he chose to, quietly carrying it.

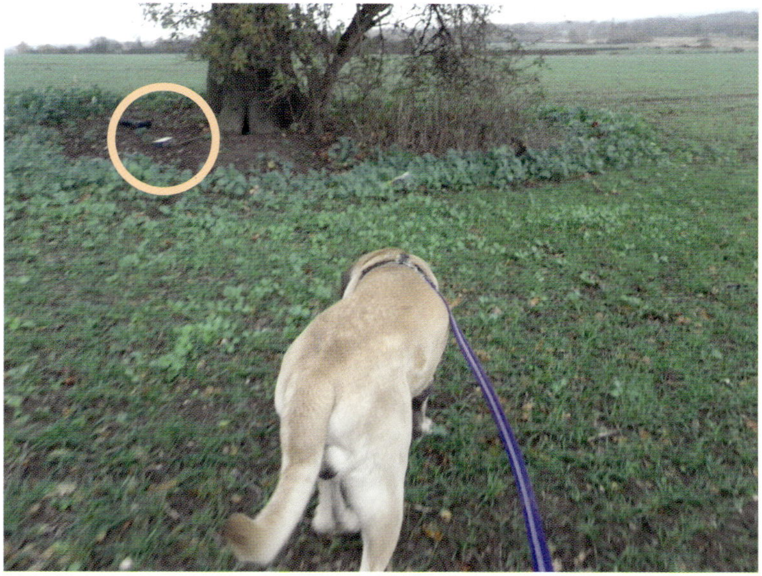

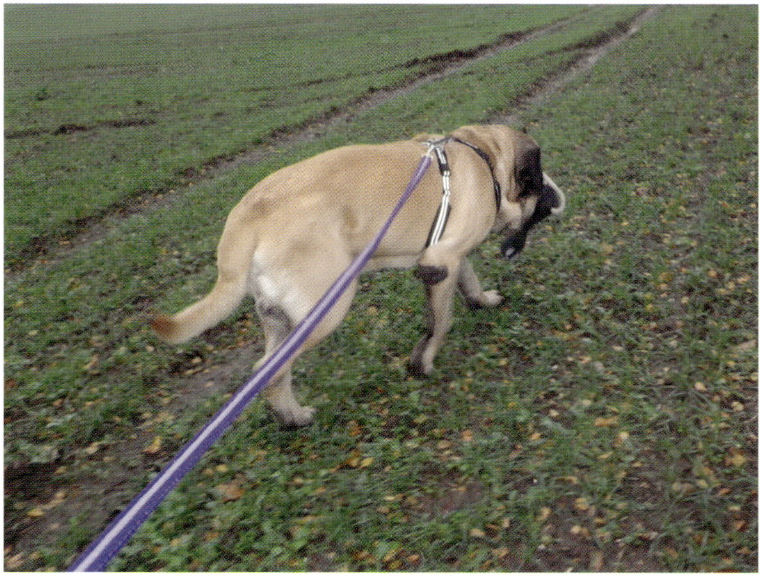

I love seeing dogs showing fulfilment in their own way, which of course is in contrast to how I first thought they did. I've learned to see and appreciate genuine pleasure in dogs, expressed in their own way, not always in the way many might expect.

It's my view that they don't need to be subjected to these standards, and if they are, it often has a negative effect on them because generally they have a different natural pace of life. It's a personal choice, but important to be aware of the damage that could be done. I'd like to gently put the emphasis back on enjoyment and learning at a natural pace.

If Hagrid didn't find his toys on a walk, it didn't matter to me if he missed one or found other scents more interesting and, as far as he showed, it didn't matter to him either. However, it is important for some dogs if they don't find what they're looking for; they may become frustrated.

Occasionally, when Hagrid was looking for a toy, after a while, I'd give him gentle and subtle guidance, ensuring he was the one who found it and not me, and then next time I might make it easier. This could have been an example of me having made it too difficult that time, weather conditions, wind direction, him not being able to concentrate, or finding something else more interesting. I also found that when Hagrid was too excited, it would be detrimental to his experience. He'd go off track and not be able to focus properly.

The point is, there are many reasons why a dog could lose the scent, but it doesn't matter so much, as long as they're enjoying themselves and not frustrated; that's the real goal.

Drawing parallels

There are many instances when parallels can be drawn between children and dogs. I use these analogies because I think it's interesting to notice the similarities and, I hope, easier to understand from a human point of view.

I've used the photos opposite because of the parallel with dogs finding 'treasure' on walks.

The children explored and interacted with what they'd come across because it was a chance for them to build their skills in a supervised way. In future, and if in a similar situation, they'd understand how to use a saw safely and know the dangers involved.

They were given choices, and when it's of their choosing, it sets the scene for learning to take place. If I'd have said 'no' it could have detracted from their natural curiosity, prevented a learning opportunity, and damaged their self-confidence.

When we took the treasure bags out of the truck at home, Pogo also found them highly interesting, rifling through bits of the rubbish. Although once a highly tense little dog, she was now in a position to freely enjoy searching through the bags without coming to any harm.

She's learnt a lot about life.

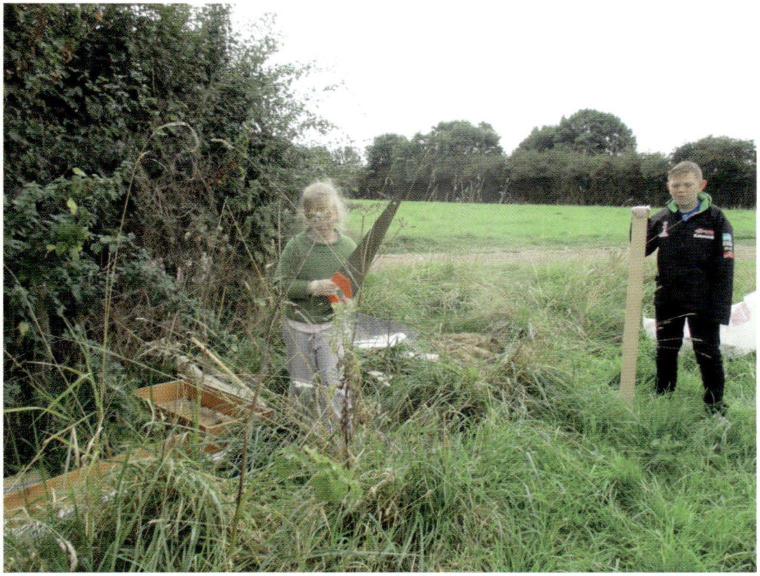

Armed with gloves and recycling bags, Katey, William and I headed off to clear a local field of litter. Earlier that day, while walking Hagrid and Pogo, we'd come across the rubbish that had been there for a week or so.

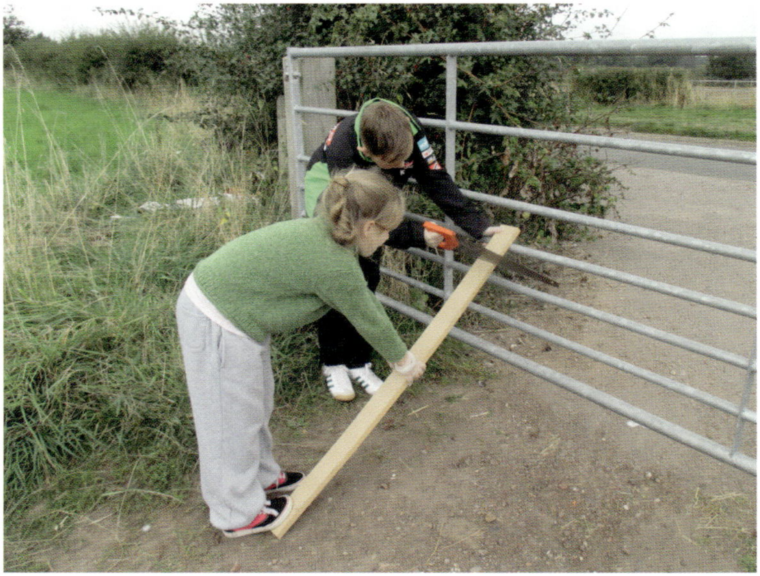

As you can see, the children found the litter quite entertaining and were creative with what they found! They took it in turns to saw up wood (supervised by me of course!). The experience was enriching and helped them build some life skills in a way that was also fun and confidence building.

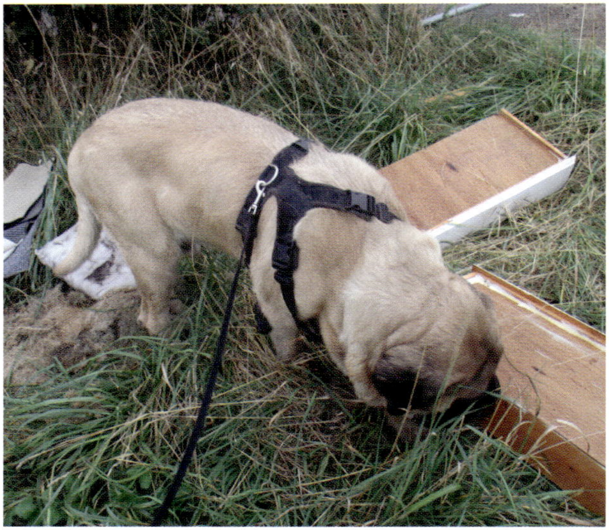

Hagrid returns to where the rubbish was dumped a few days after we'd been handling the items.

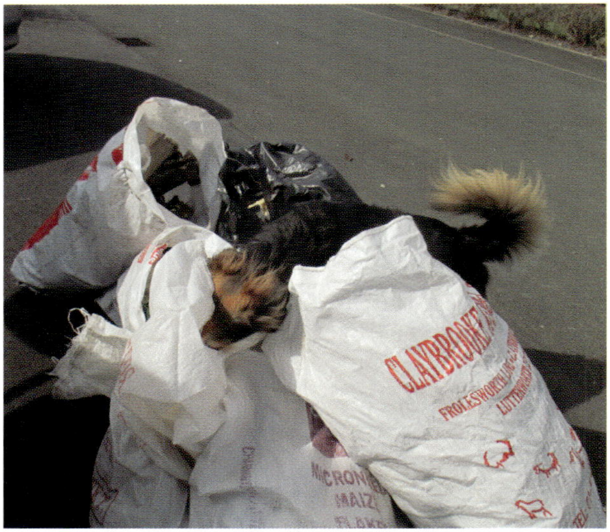

Pogo inspecting the day's pickings, which gave her so much fun. My dogs love having chances to explore.

Although Hagrid had been to the same spot a few times before the children had been there, he found the rubbish even more engaging when we visited the area a few days later. He took particular interest in going through drawers, cushions and other things left behind. Seeing his interest and how absorbed he was on this occasion made me wonder if this was because we'd spent so much time going over the items with the children. It's not a bad idea to recreate a similar, safe situation that is simple to set up, rewarding, of interest for a dog and can be cleared away afterwards.

We can learn much from observing as dogs explore. Do they want to explore? How do they go about it? Are they more adventurous when their carer is close by? How is it different when using a long-line? There's so much to learn from dogs.

Playful, relaxed learning

A bit of frustration is an inevitable part of life. Sometimes this can be character building, but an animal who becomes overly frustrated may eventually become distressed, or even give up if a task is too complicated. This in turn knocks their confidence, which is not what we're aiming for. Dogs can be overwhelmed by too much enrichment, so it needs to be carefully thought out to match his skill levels. For example, a dog who is focused on balls or other items wouldn't benefit from them being included. It would simply cause anxiety. On the other hand, suitable enrichment can add to his confidence and self-esteem, promoting an inquisitive character and stimulating brain development.

Some may choose to have a quick look as they pass new things in the environment. It's sensible to do that, but could also be that the dog is worried. By having the support of a lead, they may backtrack to have another look, before feeling it's okay to investigate further. A few may stand and stare for quite a while, unable to break their gaze. This can happen when something is too close for them. At that point, they may become reactive and could require some help from us.

With Hagrid, I could often avoid these times by intervening gently in some way such as moving a step away, or speaking kindly to him to distract his thoughts enough for him to break away. Intervention can also be carried out *before* the dog begins to become excitable. I note the distance in relation to my dog and the object, so that next time a similar situation occurs, there's a possibility to increase the gap until they are far enough away to feel at ease.

As always it's good to be mindful of their body language and communication.

Jumping up at, or looking to, the carer for support, delaying by sniffing somewhere else, or going back to check things out and urinating more frequently may accompany exploration. It may indicate that his skills need developing and if the dog has a nervous character, he could be worried by the sudden change in environment, so this is not suitable for some of them and they need more support.

Again, less is more. I say that a lot in this book because it's something I believe in. Starting with just one or two items and observing the dog's interest is appropriate.

Key points

- It's a delicate balance; some stimulation to help with enjoyment and quality of life, but not too much for a dog to become obsessive or exhausted. Less really is more.
- Just a tiny bit of help from us is needed sometimes, and in a subtle way.
- A dog needs to feel satisfied to be able to build confidence.
- I like to put the emphasis on enjoyment and learning at a natural pace.
- Intervention can be carried out before the dog begins to become excitable.

Chapter 12

Animals, vets and carers working together

This is an emotional chapter and begins with a deeply moving personal experience with the premature loss of my much loved Kaos.

I'd like to begin by saying how much most vets help our pets and are in the profession because they're dedicated to treating animals. They have an incredibly difficult job because they're not just dealing with the pets, it's the people as well. People are passionate about their pets and emotions are often close to the surface. Vets are pretty amazing if you think about it, with limited time and information about their clients, just a small window of opportunity to assess what's going on for the animal and human, and how they can help. I wonder if the animal can sometimes be the easiest part of the relationship.

When it comes to drugs being involved then the vet obviously knows more, so I rely on their expertise. With the vet's information and training, together with my knowledge and experience, we explore the best possible outcome for the animal. I look into the side effects of prescribed drugs and consider what my feelings are for them in regards to the dog. During any treatment plan I observe how my animals are. The websites I reference for information are reputable veterinary sites that are trustworthy; if there are queries about drugs I'll contact my vet and we'll discuss it.

I consider this being careful in the same way I'd search for side effects for personal medication before taking it, and ingredients listed on food packets. Some ingredients can really irritate my stomach, affect my mood and the way I think. My doctor wouldn't know that, but I would. In all professions, mistakes can happen and I want to make sure there's minimal risk for my animals.

I once had a very unfortunate experience at the vet with Kaos, my previous Mastiff. I'd been to the same vet for years, and all was well until things went so wrong. Kaos lost her life, alone at the vets; she was just five years old. It was only a routine surgery, but knowing that she died alone, away from me, grieved me more than anything. For that reason, it was time to find another surgery where there was onsite care for overnight patients to prevent the same thing happening again.

On the day of Kaos's routine operation I took her to the vet. She was given a pre-med and then I went with her to the kennel. The operation was due to take place on the same morning. Later that day the vet called to say they had been unable to perform the operation as Kaos had become too heavily sedated with just the pre-med and so I took her home.

I'd never seen a dog so out of it but took her back the next day as asked. I did question whether Kaos was okay for the operation: she still seemed to be quite affected from the previous day's pre-med. After another pre-med the operation went ahead.

The day after the surgery, I was planning to collect Kaos early in the morning. I had already visited the previous evening after the vet called to say she was ready to be picked up. However, when I'd arrived at the vet's, I was then told she'd be better off staying overnight, just to make sure all was well.

Although I questioned this and asked to bring her home anyway, I was told she should have been more awake by the time I'd arrived to collect her. I assured the vet I'd be able to attend to Kaos' needs at home and even though I stated this a couple of times, that wasn't what they wanted me to do, so I was persuaded she'd be better off with a vet close at hand in case there were problems during the night.

On my way to fetch Kaos early in the morning after, Jaffa and I had just finished a lovely walk. My mobile phone rang. My husband, Colin, phoned to say he had some awful news. I said 'no, not Kaos?' in disbelief, sensing it was connected to her. Colin confirmed it was, and told me she'd died early in the morning, alone.

As you might imagine I was distraught, as most people would be. A couple of hours later, after gathering my composure, I went with Jaffa to the vets to see Kaos' body. The vet informed me that Kaos could stay with them for a few days and my family and I could visit her whenever we liked, providing I called in advance. But when I called the vet later in the afternoon to drop in on my way home, I was horrified to find that she'd gone to be cremated without my knowledge or permission. I hadn't even decided where to have her cremated and had been told she'd remain at the vet's for a few days!

> Kaos' death was both traumatic and heart wrenching, and still is now when I think about it. Big mistakes were made.

There was no apology, although four months later I received a letter. It stated 'no charge'. I wanted to report the incident, though going over it then was just too distressing and was for a long time afterwards. A week after, the vet who performed the surgery and I discussed matters at length. He seemed transparent about everything, genuinely empathic and concerned about what had happened. I do think mistakes were made and I understand everyone makes them.

Acepromazine was used as the pre-med and this was the reason for Kaos becoming so sleepy. A different vet told me that great care needs to be taken when using this particular sort of pre-med on large breed dogs. I later found out that sedation in giant breeds can last for 12-24 hours rather than the 3-4 hours expected for a smaller dog, so now I always ask what anaesthetics are going to be used and research them first.

Another vet, a friend, has told me that certainly much more time for recovery between the pre-meds would have been advisable. I wonder if that's what killed Kaos, but I'll never know because her body was taken away less than 24 hours after her death.

What upset me the most was Kaos dying alone, somewhere she didn't want to be. It made me feel so bad leaving her there that night when I knew she wanted to come home. I'll never forget seeing her tail wagging as she recognised me when I went to pick her up the night before she died, when I wasn't allowed to take her home.

There were certainly things I would do differently now. Firstly, I would never leave a dog alone at night without a vet or anyone present. Secondly, I'd check pre-meds and anaesthetics were all suitable for the breed and individual dog. This is something I once considered to be down to the vet, but the responsibility also lies with the carer to check, as they know the dog better than anyone. It needs to be a joint effort, and this is why I try to have more input into my pets' care. It may be irritating to a few people, but someone has to stand up for the dogs' rights, and I have found many vets are willing to support and adapt to a client's wishes.

Our new vet, Graham

One of my jobs when I was a petsitter was to take clients' dogs to the vets and that's how I met Graham, our new vet. He had a pleasant approach with dogs, they liked him, he was gentle and thoughtful, and answered questions I had.

Before Graham met Hagrid, I arranged a visit on my own to explain what I wanted from a vet and also briefly mentioned my previous experience with Kaos, saying I'd changed practices because of this. This can be important for the vet to find out your background and intention before bringing any animals in. It's a chance to get to know and talk together.

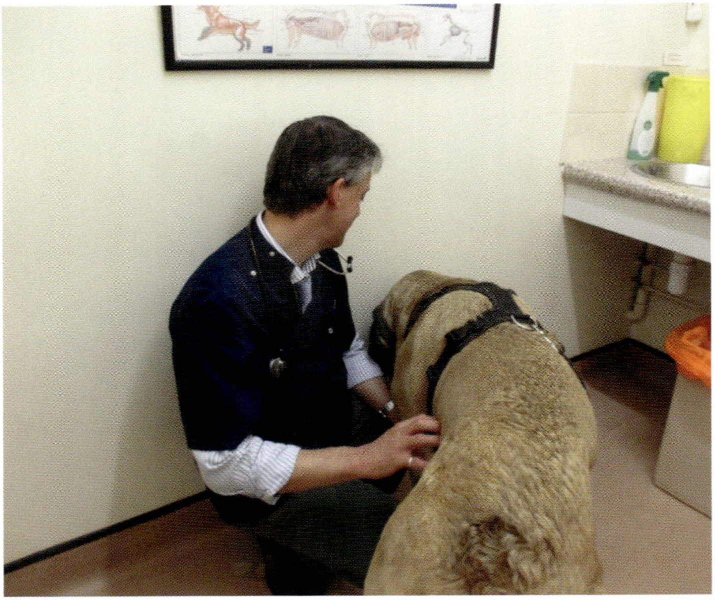

It's great that Graham gave Hagrid the opportunity to explore the room and sniff around before squatting down, giving signals to Hagrid that he was about to be touched. Being relaxed and taking his time helped Hagrid accept that something was about to happen.

As with the previous vet, I asked for things I felt were in the best interests of my dogs, even though the vet - including Graham - didn't always agree with my views. We at least discussed options, however, and he appeared to be very open and honest.

Hagrid's relationship with vets really improved because of Graham's calm approach. He was brilliant for Hagrid because he gave him time to adapt to his surroundings while we talked about his health. While doing his job, he was careful not to force Hagrid. He would always go slowly with him and had great body language – bending down, careful not to have direct eye contact.

Hagrid, like many dogs who have issues trusting people, often found eye contact overwhelming, especially when it was direct. It can quickly become intense, and in my experience dogs find it scarier the longer it continues. This could, however, be different if it's eye contact with someone they know and trust.

At the point of it becoming too intense, Hagrid would air snap, which meant he was worried, as well as it being scary for people. When I could, I'd ask the person to look away, change the situation or I'd walk in between.

Hagrid would stay close to someone and unnaturally still before air snapping. I've seen similar behaviour in other Mastiffs. They can keep an eye on a particular person and stay very close to them. It's often mistaken as a dog liking someone or that they feel safe near them, which is of course one reason for doing that. But it could also be insecurity: the need to keep the person nearby because they don't trust them. Taking these things into account, and the dog's body language, will make things clearer.

Being at the vets brings sights, sounds, touch and smells that dogs may not usually come across. These new experiences may be frightening for them and having a carer who's calm and supportive gives dogs a sense of security.

Most dogs whose behaviour seems to be good at the vet will more than likely be suppressing their emotions, and it's easy to abuse this and invade them.

The first time Hagrid went to see Graham he'd been with us for just eight days. The next time I contacted the surgery was after three weeks when we decided phone calls would be a good idea, now and then, so as not to put Hagrid under undue distress. The first step to help Hagrid regain trust was to inform my vet that Hagrid might bite, which Graham sensed anyway. I mentioned Hagrid was very nervous around people, and more so men. I'd seen that he would cower and run away. Besides, a dog in an unfamiliar place, unable to escape, may feel the need to defend themselves if they feel threatened.

In the small consulting room, Hagrid was unable to escape. Graham, being kind and gentle, didn't touch him for the first few visits, neither did he give him treats to lure him into a false sense of security because this can ultimately lead to a dog suppressing their feelings, being confused, overwhelmed in a new setting and losing trust in us. This gave Hagrid time to build up trust in people again. I would hold him in certain positions while Graham examined him at a distance. Over time, as Hagrid became more at ease with people, Graham was able to work in a more hands-on way.

I always tried to err on the side of caution when deciding if a visit to the vet was necessary, as I would with any dog. After all, it may not be a pleasant experience for them. That said, plenty can be done to make the experience as smooth for them as possible.

How I tried to make vet visits comfortable

Years ago, when I first became conscious of how important it was for my dogs to have a good relationship with the vet, I would take them to the surgery at a quiet time without an appointment. Back then, I was in 'training mode' so was eager to get them into the waiting room. My focus was on what happened inside the surgery rather than the whole experience; something I see with quite a few dog carers. I was proud of my dogs and wanted to show them off so others would give them attention. That's really not so important to a dog.

Now I realise that what happens outside the vets is valuable settling-in time for dogs, and think about the experience from their point of view. They adjust to the situation by sniffing around and gaining information. That's what's really important to them. Inside, vets and nurses will pet the dogs, focusing on them. Instead of doing this, I've learned to make the event more casual and defused, without the treats and attention from the staff. I can see this has helped my dogs accept the whole veterinary experience and the procedures far more easily, also they've seemed much more at ease being there. The whole situation is simply much calmer and more natural.

I've found that praise and attention usually makes a dog excitable and animated, often causing them to pant, setting their expectations up for something to happen, putting them on alert, so they are less able to concentrate on their surroundings or make sense of things. It's like trying to have a conversation when there's loud music. The dog needs to have the opportunity to take in his environment and go at his pace.

In my experience, turning a vet visit into a non-event can be very successful.

> Drawing attention to a vet visit can create overstimulation, which can make a dog suspicious of our behaviour and be detrimental to keeping them relaxed and grounded.

A dog that's less stressed is:

- Less of a threat to the vet.
- In a better position to give clear communication.
- Able to develop confidence.
- More aware of what to expect next time.
- Equipped to make appropriate choices.
- Aware of his surroundings.
- In a position to recover well from illness.
- Able to think more clearly.
- Easier for the vet to work with.

Graham, the vet we visited, was several miles away from us, so we travelled by van with Hagrid in the back. On arriving, he'd stay where he was while I registered at the reception. Then I'd wait with him in the van where we could see each other through the grating, until we were called in. Graham would often come outside to fetch us, which gave him an opportunity to see Hagrid walk and his general state.

Hagrid was given time. He sniffed the bushes in the car park and sometimes would have a wee before going through a side entrance to the consulting rooms. Going that way meant we didn't have to go past other dogs in the waiting area, which generally don't have the distance most animals need from each other. Dogs would usually be worried by Hagrid, so giving them space prevented putting any of them under pressure. Going to the vet is usually enough for any dog without being worried by other dogs as well.

Once in the consulting room, Graham and I would talk as Hagrid looked around and settled where he wanted, while still on his long line for support. Graham would do what he needed to, while I held Hagrid and talked to him. It isn't just about building trust between the dog and the vet, it's also a case of establishing what you're capable of and that you're prepared to be there for your dog. The best person to support a dog is usually the carer, just as children prefer their parents' company when they're not feeling well. It aids their recovery.

My dogs would need some opportunity to sniff around the area after they'd seen the vet, then I'd take them back to the van so they were nicely relaxed, before going back into the building to pick up medication, if needed, and pay. I believe this approach might be best for most dogs, providing they're happy being in the car or outside with someone they know.

After the consultation we'd go straight home. This is what suited Hagrid best, especially in the last couple of years of his life. When he was younger, a short walk somewhere familiar afterwards was an enjoyable activity, but as he got older, going home and sleeping helped him more. I'd try to make sure I was around for him after we'd been to the vet because my being around was reassuring for him.

Allowing Hagrid to have this time, without pressure, meant he could accept what was happening and adjust to it at his pace. When any animal feels as though there's a choice they are more likely to cooperate than resist. If I'd attempted to use coercion or rush him, he would have been more likely to go on the defensive. People can act in similar ways when under pressure. This is a fantastic lesson to learn, and it puts the dog in control of their situation. Obviously they need to go in, but just a bit of time can make such a big difference.

Ultimately, by taking this approach they will build up respect for you. However, the animal needs to be given the time to trust first to make decisions in their lives, and every animal will have their own pace.

We took this protocol with us to each vet visit, even on the more important visits when there were emergencies and/or operations due. I always asked the vet to give Hagrid time to settle in the room before receiving any hands-on treatment, also requesting that I stayed with him at all times if possible.

The skin specialist vet, Richard Harvey

Before an operation with a specialist vet, Richard Harvey, Hagrid remained in the van while Colin and I went to speak to the consultant. I was able to state what Hagrid's needs were, and came away feeling this had been a positive experience.

Prior to the operation, Richard and I discussed if I could be with Hagrid until he was under anaesthetic, as well as when he came round afterwards. There was a bit of uncertainty, but both vets involved worked out a way to accommodate us. It ran seamlessly and Richard was great at finding ways around their protocols so I could be with Hagrid until he'd been sedated.

Richard had a speedy manner but made compromises while Hagrid explored his surroundings. Richard

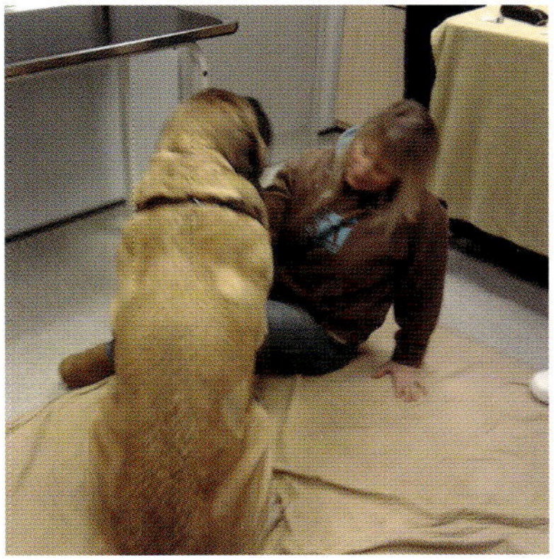 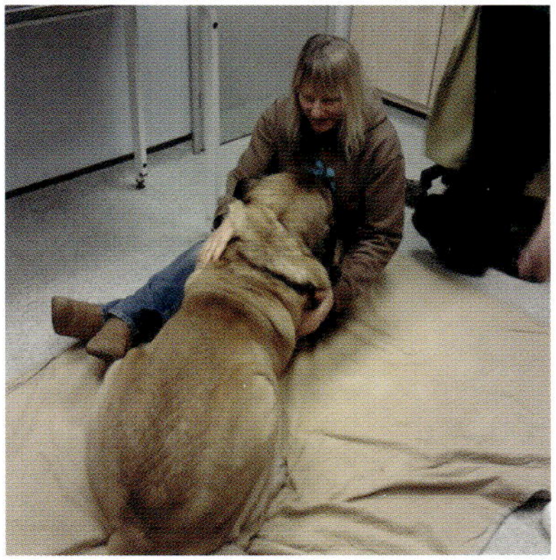 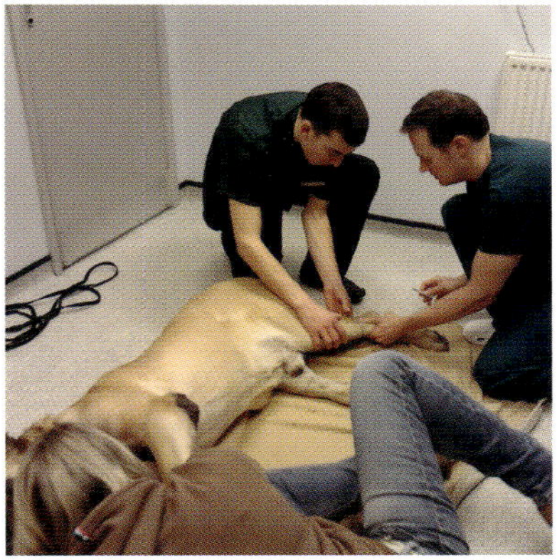

For any dog that experiences an operation, it must be traumatic. Here, vet Conor and vet nurse Martin at Godiva vet in Coventry, carry out the pre-med on Hagrid. Once unconscious, Hagrid was wrapped in the blanket he sat on and we all lifted him onto a trolley. Staying with Hagrid, emotionally and physically supporting him through this experience at the vets was crucial. We as carers can make such a difference to an animal's experience.

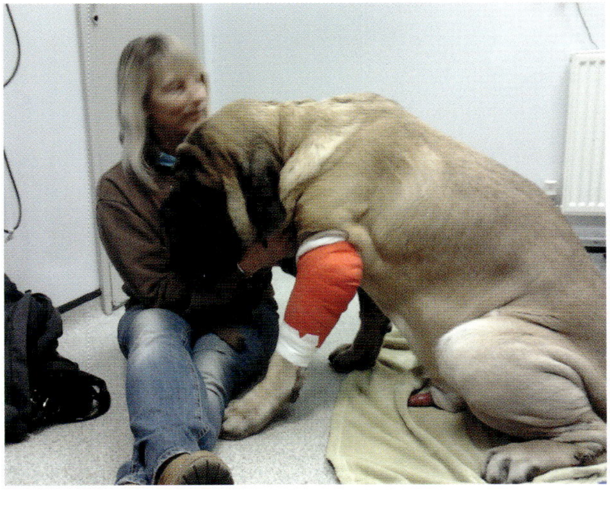 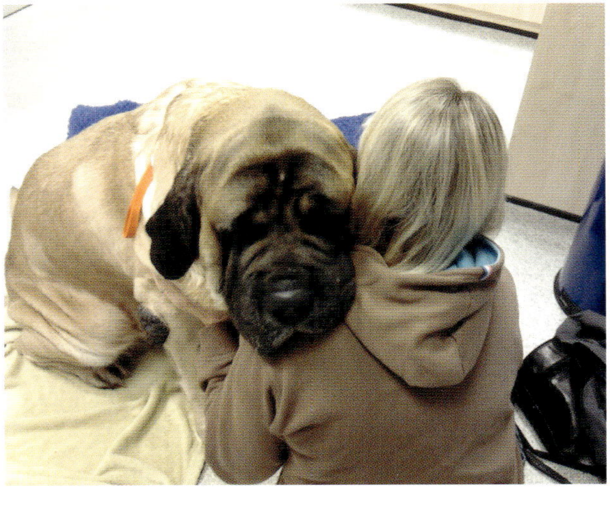

began his investigations and Hagrid was fine with him; he was so relaxed in there and even felt comfortable enough to lie down without panting or being tense. With all that completed, we put Hagrid back in the van. I'd never seen him so relaxed in a vet's examination room.

Everything went well on the morning of the operation. We were with Hagrid until he was fully sedated, then all four of us lifted the blanket Hagrid was on onto the operating trolley.

Colin and I went across the road and sat in a café while the procedure took place. When Hagrid was just coming round from the anaesthetic, Richard came over to the café to fetch us so I was able to sit with Hagrid until he'd fully regained consciousness and was ready to leave. What a positive experience for all.

Experience with the homeopathic vet, Christopher Day

The first time we visited the homeopathic vet Christopher Day, none of us knew what to expect. It was a tense time, with a two-hour drive and it was a hot summer's day, temperatures exceeding 27 degrees. Hagrid struggled in the heat, so we took plenty of water with us and parked in a shady spot.

On reaching the vet's room, we had a pleasant experience; Chris was great, slow and took his time. Both Hagrid and Jaffa were able to explore all of his office, while we sat and the vet took a full history of the dogs. It was a holistic approach, and we learnt ways of improving home life for the dogs; being aware of the effects of cleaning products, perfumes and smells in the house, the impact of different vessels for the dogs to drink and eat out of and much more.

Having previously visited Chris with Kaos, we already knew several ways to enhance a dog's life (and ours) by making small lifestyle changes. We were able to take this to another stage to improve life for all of us by following his recommendations.

Chris's room was excellent for the dogs on such a steaming hot day. It was in an old house with a flagstone floor, and very fresh. Hagrid and Jaffa sprawled out on it and as they were given lots of time while the vet explained about areas we could work on, the dogs were cooled down and relaxed.

It was such a great way to do business, to see the dogs naturally because he simply observed from his desk. They were relaxed and had freedom to wander around the room. Before we left for home the dogs were rested and refreshed. We loved Chris's hands-off approach and so did our dogs.

This experience contrasted sharply with a visit to another vet...

Near the end of Hagrid's life

Hagrid had become very ill and was on painkillers that had been increased over the days before. The pain he was experiencing was significant, and although an appointment was booked, the situation had deteriorated, requiring an emergency trip to our vet before going straight to the specialist vet. Hagrid had required further pain medication, and without visiting a specialist vet, no more could be done; he was incredibly poorly. Colin was away on business, so I went alone.

The whole visit, although necessary for further treatment, was most distressing for both of us. But more so for Hagrid, and this heavily impacted on his last few weeks of life.

Although Hagrid had been getting progressively worse, after that day his quality of life was severely compromised. I was Hagrid's advocate, and no one knew him better. I wish I'd taken up the offer of my colleague Sheila Harper's support when she made it. Sheila had made this kind offer the day before, when I called her to talk options through. At the time though, I knew she had a lot on her plate and so decided to go alone with a view to standing up for what was right for Hagrid. Above all, I knew he needed me with him and although I did my best at the time to assert this, I was unable to carry out my intentions.

After two hours of questioning me about Hagrid's health and history, putting him through various physical manipulations and walking up and down corridors with him, the vet was ready to take blood from Hagrid, who had just that second lain down for the first time right near the door. He had been panting the whole time. The vet said he needed to take some blood and I actually said, "You're joking." I couldn't believe what I'd just heard. Didn't he realise the impact on Hagrid of the past two hours? He said Hagrid would need to go with him to the next room to have blood taken. I asked if he could instead take blood from him as he was, lying on the floor. We'd done this numerous times with previous vets, and all was absolutely fine. In fact, no one had ever asked to take any of my animals out of the room to take blood from them. The vet said they needed to go into the next room and owners weren't allowed in.

I'd phoned ahead of the visit and stated Hagrid's need for me to be with him and that had been agreed, but now this vet insisted owners weren't allowed to go into the next room: there are other patients in there and that they'd only be five minutes.

Again I stressed Hagrid's need for me to be with him, asking if blood could be taken in the room we were in. The vet refused and said they'd be back in five minutes before taking Hagrid away to the next room.

For me, remembering this, even writing this, is so painful and I recall how it felt to let Hagrid go.

Like so many others, I find challenging authority frightening, though still possible. Our life's conditioning can prevent us from speaking up for what we need, and although I did speak up, I didn't turn around and walk out with Hagrid because he needed pain killers and I believed this was the only way for Hagrid to be out of pain now.

Three cups of tea and half an hour later, the vet and an exhausted Hagrid came back into the room: this was most definitely not the five minutes I'd been promised. I'd never seen Hagrid's tongue swell so much: it was lolling out of the side of his mouth. He was so, so distressed. I asked to put him back into the van at that point, but the vet said I'd have to wait until after he'd told me his findings. Can you imagine the distress?

Hagrid wasn't even able to lie down at this point, and I could see how worried he was. Of course, I couldn't hear much of what the vet said at that moment, because my concern and attention was on Hagrid and my disbelief at the situation.

What I did understand (and won't forget) was the vet saying how great it was to see Hagrid in the outside area, off-lead. WHAT?! My brain froze. I knew Hagrid could never be off-lead outside because his lack of awareness caused him to be bewildered, worried and perplexed. The vet told me how he'd stumbled and fallen several times and walked into the fence. I knew this would have caused Hagrid great anxiety.

Where was the empathy for my dog? My Hagrid. This was cruelty! I would never let him off lead for these very reasons and had already informed the vet of this. We'd walked up and down the corridor (Hagrid being guided on-lead) at least four times at the vet's request, and that had been heartbreaking already to see Hagrid falling, aimlessly wandering, expecting to walk out of the building each time we headed in the direction of the exit.

Not only that, I'd also supplied the vet with plenty of video footage of Hagrid walking off-lead outside in the garden where he felt safe and knew his surroundings. There was no need for the vet to have done that, especially when he'd reassured me that all he would be doing would be taking some blood.

I was told the vet and his colleagues had been able to watch Hagrid outside, aimlessly wandering around bumping into fences, knuckling (falling on his wrist joints) and having no awareness. How distressing when he didn't understand what was going on, didn't know anyone and was in an unfamiliar environment. How could anyone do this without seeing his obvious distress? What had they done to Hagrid, without my consent, which I would never have given? We had to get out, but I still needed to get further pain medication; the whole reason for us being there.

While there are many, obviously caring and empathetic vets, this one really had no empathy for my dog at all. He was clinical, but there's far more to his job than that. Vision and compassion were necessary and most definitely missing on that day. Without a doubt, Hagrid was nearing the end of his life, and now I wondered if he'd survive what he'd just experienced.

Changing attitudes

I see dogs are repeatedly ignored through lack of understanding and this must be so distressing for them. Imagine how it would feel to have your attempts at communication ignored by those around you.

There were times not so long ago when children would be hospitalised and their parents could visit within restricted times but weren't allowed to stay with them. Imagine what those children must have felt like when their parents left them alone at a time when they were ill, vulnerable and needed their comfort and support.

This approach to medical care was thankfully brought to an end with the realisation that there was a faster recovery rate if parents stayed with their children.

> Being cared for and the feeling of being cared for is incredibly important for any animal, especially one that's unwell.

While it's possible to explain things to children, animals don't understand what's happening to them. Wouldn't it be better if they were able to have the support of their carer - someone they know and trust? It could prove to be as beneficial for their recovery as it is for children having their parents with them.

I've been told so many times that my dog will misbehave if I stayed with them at the vets; it would be much better for them and they'd be better behaved if they're left alone. But this happens because dogs appear to be well behaved when really they're frightened. They're scared, vulnerable and very often hide their feelings in this situation. Staying quiet without reacting and just going along with things is viewed as good behaviour.

This kind of emotional shutting down doesn't just happen at the vets; it can and does happen in many places, for example; when they're left to be groomed, at day care centres, boarding kennels and so on. It can even take place at home and when they're left with someone to look after them.

Being able to express emotions is such a positive and healthy sign, although sometimes it can be a little against what we would ideally want, and maybe we feel embarrassed. Showing emotions is positive for mental wellness and physical health. And if we know how an animal is feeling, it's possible to make adaptations and help them feel more comfortable, although this can mean more work for us.

There might be signs of the release of this stress afterwards as well, such as being incredibly excited to be reunited with their carer, urination, and drinking lots, among others. I've known my dogs to be ecstatic when collecting them from somewhere and it felt nice at the time, for me, that they were so pleased to see me.

Imagine you're in a foreign country and find yourself left with people you don't know. You are dealing with unfamiliar people, unable to communicate with them, you don't speak their language and don't understand their customs or culture, which vary from country to country. The wrong communication signals can lead to misunderstanding and trouble. In this situation, you would probably be quite subdued for fear of what might happen.

The canine equivalent at the vets can be similar - the environment is very different from what the dog is used to; he's surrounded by distressed and ill animals, some making upsetting noises, as well as the many smells that go with treatment and illness. Then ultimately he has procedures performed that are invasive, possibly painful, and are against his will.

I'm aware that plenty of pets do recover from surgery and other procedures, but things can be so much better if their communication were to be taken into account, they were understood and listened to. We need to adopt more of an animal-centred approach.

A few of my animals have suffered from the way they were dealt with and how procedures were carried out. I wonder how many people are scarred, as I am. Even though things have been done in a certain way for all our lives, does that make it right? I'm sure there is room for improvement and have worked with vets who can make simple yet effective changes to accommodate animals' needs.

Having written this chapter, I was pleasantly surprised when a colleague brought to my attention the work of Rebekah Hudson from America, who shares some of the same beliefs, that change for animals while at the vet is necessary for their well-being.

The good news is, it's starting to take place.

I have included links to Rebekah's site, and some other select studies into animal well-being at the end of the chapter.

A good vet is someone who:

- The animal likes and feels comfortable with.
- Listens to both carer and animal.
- Takes their time.
- Has a gentle manner with the animal.
- Discusses options rather than dictating treatment plans.
- Doesn't simply push conventional ideas and will explore alternative health solutions.
- Treats you as an equal and gives you respect.

Finding a good vet

Through my work with dogs I've often heard people talk about a good vet. 'I've found a good vet'. But every time I hear it, I wonder what it means. When asking friends about their views, some different ideas arose. So here's a sample of what they shared.

I understand that this is a lot to expect from one person! Really I'm looking for the closest possible match, and prioritising the most important factors for the particular animal going to the vet.

When it came to deepening the understanding of what a good vet is, I started by considering how I would go about finding a new vet if I needed to.

What struck me was how many factors have to come into consideration. Firstly, the practicalities are essential. For example, the building itself, its size, where the doors are, and what options my animals will have to go in and come out. In other words, how many entrances are there? Would it be possible to park in the shade, away from others if necessary?

Other practical considerations include the waiting area. How are they set up for different animals and is there space for them to be away from each other without having to react and be worried? Can each species have a section away from the others?

Another consideration is accessibility. The car park and outdoor areas are vital for dogs to be able to explore before and after they're in the vets. When a dog is under pressure they'll need to urinate and defecate more frequently, so it's important to make sure there's a good space for this. Mentally, I plan my route in and out of the surgery, and also consider the backup options if there isn't a free car parking space. How far would I have to walk with a potentially distressed dog?

The surrounding environment also ties into this. Some vet buildings might be unsuitable because they're on a busy main road. This could be unsafe for some nervous dogs, though for others it could be fine. Consider the nature of the animal and how they may respond to different environments.

I've mainly found veterinary teams to be very friendly, professional and welcoming. It certainly helps me to feel at ease, and that's passed on to the animal. The nature of the reception and nursing staff, the management, as well as the vet, all contribute to the overall feel of the environment. This is something I can instinctively pick up on.

Before taking an animal to see the vet I like to visit without my dogs, to get a sense of what the morale and atmosphere is like. Did it feel comfortable? Was I welcomed? How were my questions answered? Was I listened to respectfully? Being allowed to stay with a dog through procedures is a topic to discuss in advance with a vet.

Having lost a dog, possibly due to incorrect administration of anaesthetics, I would tell them about my previous experiences so they can understand the background to any queries I might have and my general attitude towards animal well-being. I would want to know about the types of drugs used and receive this information prior to anything being administered.

The medical world has vastly changed over recent years, with more and more practitioners accepting the value of a holistic approach. Many vets are open to this. A vet who is unbiased to the benefits of natural, integrated healthcare is someone I would want to choose.

Finding a vet who is relaxed, has a calm approach, and who is willing to give my dogs time to adjust to their surroundings is most important for me. This, in turn, gives time to settle in before anything happens. Building trust is a great investment from the animal's point of view. I also like a more hands-off approach where possible, especially in the early days, and prefer a vet who is willing to listen and work with me to gain the best result for the animal, meaning that they would respect and consider my choices, particularly about complementary therapies. It's part of the vet's job to be fluent in their communication with clients and is more likely that instructions will be carried out if the client understands clearly how to administer medication.

I would appreciate honesty too and for the vet to say in their opinion if specific procedures were likely to be too invasive for the individual animal. Knowing when enough is enough and relaying that information is important. The vet and I need to make decisions together.

As part of my research for this chapter I consulted with a good friend and colleague who is a vet and she was able to provide a fresh perspective on some of my views. I find it's always positive to get another perspective. When we began to discuss how vets work, I learned that they can feel quite pressured by the amount of appointments they need to get through in a day. I hadn't realised life from their perspective was like that. There are things we can do to help make that appointment time count so that our animals get the best service.

Naturally, the communication that needs to take place takes time and most vet practices operate on a ten-minute consultation schedule. The time for a consultation doesn't really allow for much explanation! Imagine what has to be slotted into these few minutes. Getting the client and pet into the consultation room, ideally giving them some time to adjust, finding out about the issue, examining the animal, explain findings to the owner, discussing treatment options, including the possible need for further investigations and the cost for all of this, then starting the treatment.

Most vets can put the basics into these ten minutes, but anything extra becomes exceptionally tricky, and many pet owners complain that it often feels like being on a conveyer belt. One solution can be to ask if the vet is happy to provide double appointments to give that extra bit of time, but of course you may be asked to pay for this. Ultimately, it's down to the discretion of the practice as to whether they charge for this or not. It's also possible for the client to ask in advance how their particular practice works, so everyone knows up front what is involved. Despite what can seem like a hefty bill, the vast majority of vets genuinely want to do the best to help the animals.

I was interested to learn from my vet friend that some of her colleagues find it quite challenging when their customers do research online to try and diagnose what might be wrong with their animal. It's worth bearing in mind that if a client looks online, not every vet will necessarily be open to listening to that information, and that people doing that must be quite frustrating after all the years they spent training.

In my experience, people check online when they feel worried and want to understand more. If we remember the vet is likely to be on a ten-minute timeframe for each appointment, we can be more understanding and see why they might prefer to focus on making a diagnosis that is backed up by their training. As with most of the content in this book, my hope is for collaboration and equality with animal, vet and carer.

Links

Rebekah Hudson:
medium.com/@theunlikelytricksters/youll-get-used-to-it-won-t-you-179933a314c2

There are some scientific studies at the end of this article:
wherescienceanddogsmeet.wordpress.com/2018/07/06/taking-dogs-to-the-back-of-the-veterinary-clinic-why/

Some positive changes are beginning to happen at a veterinary clinic in New York, America, who actively encourage carers to stay with their pets during procedures:
veg.vet

I agree with Linda Case about vets. The Science Dog:
thesciencedog.com/2018/02/28/be-there/

Vet Amber Batson makes changes for dogs:
facebook.com/story.php?story_fbid=1362950364044636&id=131337460539272

| Chapter 13 |

Homeopathy

Homeopathy was the first alternative/complementary therapy we chose to explore for Hagrid and often, the tablets chosen were effective for a day or two. For example, the preparations gave immediate relief for the pain in his ears.

His ears would ooze and were often hot, red and sore. They would bleed from scratching and constantly shaking his head. I felt his distress as he panted, shook himself and found it hard to settle anywhere, so I would go out in the garden with him or for a walk round the block, taking our time. He would sniff and the environment offered him a chance to become absorbed with all that was available. At times that eased his symptoms or at least gave him a change of scenery for a while. The idea was to give him another focus. If humans are unwell, it can help for a while to have a distraction to take our minds off the discomfort. I know that sometimes when I'm ill I like to be outside despite the weather, instinctively feeling that's what's needed.

From keeping a diary of these and other observations, we identified a link between Hagrid's ear and skin problems and an emotional response partly caused by my being out of the house for more than a few hours. Being away for half a day was as much as he was able to deal with, despite the fact that other people he knew well would be there with him. Perhaps it was the uncertainty of what he was exposed to while I was out (such as visitors and so forth) which he found difficult.

When I was at home, I'd have boundaries in place so that he could feel safe but when I wasn't there, because he lay low and didn't react to visitors, it appeared that boundaries weren't necessary. In my view, I think he felt life was more predictable when I was around and felt secure enough to react to intrusions into his space and home environment, so was free to react when he felt anxious.

Something else that I noted from the diary; certain conditions and times of day would prompt an eruption in his ailments. Hagrid's ears would start to cause him real discomfort during the evenings, around the time we sat down to relax in the lounge, whether he was in the room with us or not. It could happen during the day too, but evenings were much more likely and noticeable.

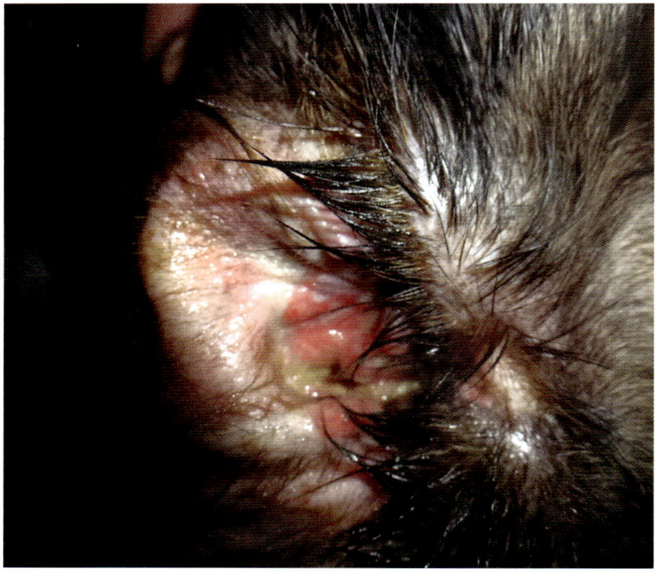

How Hagrid's ears would be, and this would often begin during the evenings.

We were sometimes able to tell if his ears would be troublesome, as one would hang down prior to a flare up. He had a specific routine when it all started to hurt; making vocal noises and rolling around; and invariably this was the cue for a 'bad ear evening'. Once he'd done that he'd seek me out for comfort. It was as if he was saying, '*please can you do something about this*?' even though he didn't use these words!

I'd massage his ears, which he visibly enjoyed. It seemed to soothe him. He'd go to Colin for the same treatment if he'd not had enough from me, or if I had left the room to fetch something. He'd then come back to me. On a good evening that might relax him but if not, it might mean that I stayed up with him for an hour or so until he could settle.

Although Hagrid was on various homeopathic remedies, Belladonna was given for these outbreaks. At first they noticeably made a difference and Hagrid would settle after around half an hour, but as time went on the positive effects wore off.

Hagrid was one for lying outside on the patio, to keep cool or sunbathe. Lying there was part of his repertoire and another indicator that his ears made him very uncomfortable. The kitchen floor was another of these cool places he'd choose to lie.

Knowing when to explore other options

Whilst some of the homeopathic remedies would make a slight difference, usually lasting for a few days or so, there were no treatments that gave significant relief, even when given over a long period of time. It appeared that homeopathy was not really working for Hagrid, so we left that behind in search of a longer-term cure. Because Hagrid's immune system was severely compromised and while all the things we did were stepping-stones to improve it, I feared that nothing would make him completely well.

This is not to say that other dogs may not benefit. There were some positive outcomes and learning that came from exploring homeopathy. These are some of the things I learned.

In an earlier chapter I introduced Christopher Day, who has been a homeopathic vet for more than thirty years and practices homeopathy as well as other therapies at his home in Oxford. He was informative, enlightening us to potential environmental factors at play in our home, which may either help or contribute to issues.

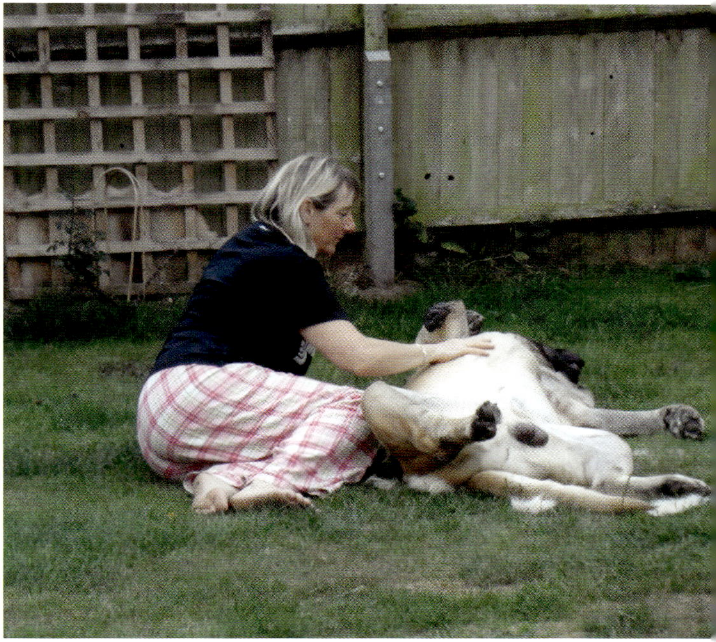

Hagrid being soothed and groomed, taking his mind off being uncomfortable.

There were little changes, mentioned in the chapter about Vets, which we made for our dogs that impacted positively on their well-being. It was reassuring to know much of what we were already doing was helping Hagrid, but there was still more we could do/explore.

I must re-emphasise how important Chris's hands-off approach and calm manner was for our dogs, in helping them to trust humans. The dogs were able to move around the room freely and get to know him as he chatted to us, sitting at his desk. He didn't attempt to fuss them, offer them treats or give them attention by way of direct eye contact or speech while he asked us relevant questions. As a result, they were soon at ease in the room and settled on the cold tiled floor.

A note on treats in a clinical setting

This is something I also mentioned in the chapter about vets, and you may be wondering why I felt it is positive that dogs aren't offered treats in this setting. It is my experience that offering a dog a treat can create a false sense of security. They are being asked to like a person, or a situation, that may not be pleasant for them. In a sense, it's bribery rather than a development or foundation for a meaningful relationship.

When treats are involved in this way, I know my dogs can become more interested in them and will therefore stop thinking clearly. Moreover, they can become more animated. Intriguingly, most people often interpret this excitement as a positive thing. However, is it fair to over excite a dog, when we have learned that children (and adults for that matter) who are overexcited can tend to make poor choices? Chris was a stranger to our dogs. And I wonder, is it fair to bribe dogs to approach strangers?

My dogs are allowed to make informed, honest decisions on whom they'd like to approach. I've known people to be bitten when trying to befriend a dog who is in conflict about going for a treat and not wanting to approach the person. It can be very dangerous.

What I learnt

The time spent with Chris was interesting and his philosophy certainly matched ours. I'd advise anyone looking out for a homeopathic practitioner to seek similar synergy.

The one or two visits throughout the months we worked with homeopathy was enough for Hagrid. Travelling to sessions and the associated stress, no matter how calming the practitioner, can affect a dog for longer than most carers realise. Each visit to any vet usually has some impact on an animal and with homeopathy that was minimised through phone contact and diary keeping.

Spacing out the appointments was an important factor in the treatment.

Although we didn't continue with homeopathy, it was useful for looking deeply at what was happening for Hagrid, as well as noticing the small changes/ improvements in him after medication. It taught us to look more closely. There were other benefits:

- We learned about the effectiveness of a hands-off approach.
- We observed the importance of taking the time to get to know the dogs and us, and how we all integrate with one another.
- Keeping a diary showed us how things were developing and progressing over time.
- The diary also enabled us to observe patterns.
- We learned about the many small environmental changes that were put into place. I strongly believe these can make a huge difference to dogs' lives.

As I've mentioned, homeopathy was good for light relief for Hagrid, but not as an overall cure. Nothing was.

And so, crucially, we learned when to accept that we had tried hard enough with one avenue of exploration and when to try something different. It was important to use my intuition to know when we'd gone as far as we could go with something.

Chapter 14

Acupuncture

Simply put, acupuncture is an ancient Chinese medicine that uses small needles placed into the body at various points. Even though needles are used, the procedure is relatively pain free. Acupuncture is often used to treat symptoms such as:

- Aches and pains
- Headaches
- Backache
- Depression / stress
- Osteoarthritis
- Digestive problems

We wondered whether this was something that might well help Hagrid with his recurring limp, something he had from an old leg injury.

At certain stages of Hagrid's life he walked with a limp, usually on the front right leg. Limping was, along with other problems, evident within the first month of him being in our home. I had the impression that prior to coming to live with us he hadn't done a lot of walking, but being with us meant he had more opportunity to do so.

The way he travelled in the van was another cause of him limping. Hagrid would like to look out of the back window to see what was going on, much to everyone's amusement. He'd rest his head on the ledge of the window and I think that when the van went around bends it caused his weight to be heavily concentrated on his front legs. Constantly being braced would put strain on them too.

Despite having very short walks, and I mean a matter of round the block - less than 400 metres, Hagrid still struggled with this limp. We found out that he'd had operations on that leg, so it was important to build exercise up slowly.

And that's what we did.

As well as resting, which meant *literally* no walks for certain periods, we introduced a very big dog crate to rule out being in the van and taking corners as a potential cause of him limping. Unfortunately though, the damage had been done.

Another intervention we made that we hoped would help was that in our house, all of our downstairs flooring had anti-slip mats for our animals' benefits. We wanted them to be able to move around safely, feel comfortable and so the wood and stone floor was covered.

Slippery floors put stresses and strains on a dog's legs, back and by implication their whole body because they have to tense in order to walk without slipping. It's important to recognise that over the long-term this can cause damage to their legs and other parts of their bodies.

Despite the mats, Hagrid still had a limp and so I looked into him having acupuncture. I discovered a place that offered this service to dogs. While having the treatment, Hagrid and I sat together for half an hour. He was not at ease and only able to settle for some of the time. It left me wondering, how beneficial a treatment is if a dog is unable to settle and accept it?

When people have acupuncture, it works best when they're relaxed. That said, we can ask for the

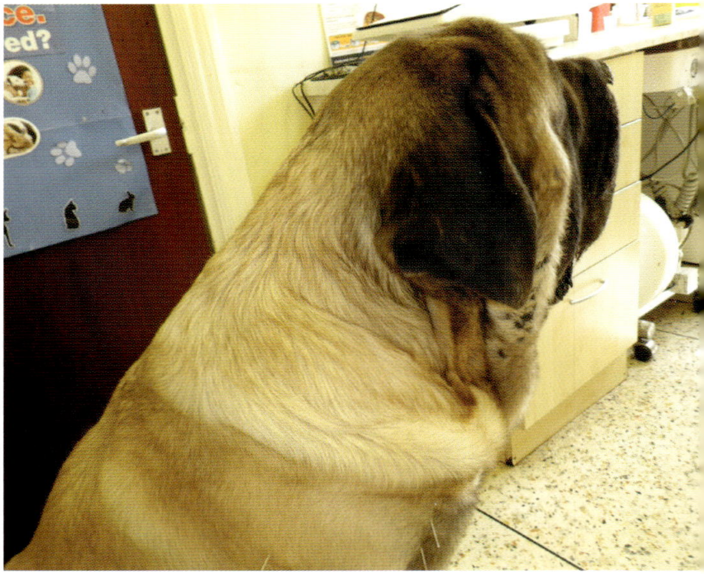

In this photo, a few acupuncture needles can be seen at the top of Hagrid's front leg.

conditions that offer the best opportunity for our dogs to be able to relax. Could there be another place for a dog to wait, while allowing the acupuncture time to work? Maybe at home or while they are in their car? Obviously this will be individual to the animal, vet and the facilities available, but it's worthwhile trying to increase the potential for success where we can.

The first acupuncturist we saw wasn't suitable because of the approach they used, even though we'd explained about Hagrid needing time to process what was happening. Although the person was nice enough and very efficient, they didn't give Hagrid time to adjust to the room before invading his space in an unsympathetic way. Their manner was hurried, which of course might be fine for some people, but not for most dogs, and it definitely didn't suit Hagrid. We felt we needed to find someone else who might be more accommodating.

Having found another practitioner, I asked for an appointment at a quiet time of the day. Hagrid stayed in the van until we went in, rather than sitting in the waiting room. At this surgery we had the option of using the front or back door, which is always a great option to have. Because no one was in the surgery (we were the last clients) and only one vet was on duty, I asked if Hagrid could be given time to become familiar with his surroundings and the surgery were happy for this to happen.

It was an opportunity for him to have some enrichment too. Other animals had been in the area and left all kinds of interesting smells. Hagrid took a minute or two to look around and was gently guided as we followed the vet into the consulting room. I'd said that he would require sensitive handling and a slow approach. After several questions were asked and answered, the vet began to place the acupuncture needles. Then she left us alone in the room for twenty minutes.

Hagrid panted a lot of the time, which in this case was a sign of stress, but he was able to explore the room freely and have choices of where to lie, all the time supported by the long line with me on the other end. Most dogs like the support of their carer, it helps them to cope with difficult situations. Having a long line gives a dog a connection with their carer and a sense of security, while still having an amount of freedom.

On this first visit, everything was new and Hagrid wasn't able to settle fully, but the second time we went he could lie down and relax more. He became a well-liked patient and although he didn't want to go into the surgery, he accepted it without fuss. He was always given choices around sniffing and weeing outside before coming in. He was allowed to come through the reception area and into the treatment room in his own time. I always stayed with Hagrid throughout his sessions and we'd leave from either the front or back door, whichever he found easiest at the time. Once the course of acupuncture had finished, it took a week or so before his limp improved. After that, Hagrid didn't limp again. But, like everything for Hagrid, there was a delayed reaction.

For this specific issue, acupuncture was successful. He needed some treatment and intervention, rather than just a few days' rest.

Recommendations for finding practitioners

There are many individual practitioners and surgeries that offer acupuncture for animals. Just as with treatments for people, it pays to research and find one who is registered, experienced and able to work specifically with the issues with which that the dog is suffering.

A good place to start is abva.co.uk. I would speak with the practitioner to find out more and explore whether the environment is right and therapeutic for my dog. If the practice is busy and my dog is either nervous or stressed, then this isn't going to be conducive to a healing experience. In fact, it might even make things worse. As I did with Hagrid, it's possible to request an appointment at the end of the working day, or during another period when they're quieter.

I gave myself plenty of time for the appointment so I was relaxed for him to be able to take his time and be at ease. Generally, if a carer is present, calm and grounded, a dog is more likely to follow their cues and feel safe. This is what I tried to do.

Physical comfort and reassurance have their place if a dog asks for it. Providing physical reassurance was important as it created calm and peace for Hagrid, done in an appropriate way for him; slowly. I was always aware of my pace and movement so that Hagrid would be likely to emulate it. Sometimes I could see he was best left alone without physical contact; being close to him and supportive was enough at the time.

While the treatment was taking place, having a more hands off approach was better. Hagrid did the communicating and I responded to his needs.

It took a few appointments before Hagrid settled into the experience and benefitted from the acupuncture itself, so we persevered. It was a real benefit to give that additional time at the start and end of the appointment to allow for a good sniff around, to let him familiarise himself with the new surroundings.

CHAPTER 15

Zoopharmacognosy: a form of self-selection and self-healing

Zoopharmacognosy is a process where a trained practitioner guides animals to select, and take in, natural compounds to reduce the harmful effects of pathogens and toxins that they may have in their systems.

It gives them the opportunity to self-medicate by offering plant extracts that would contain the same, or similar ingredients to those found in the natural environment.

While being monitored, self-selection sets the scene for the animal to guide its own health; unlike their wild counterparts, captive and domesticated animals rarely have the chance seek out appropriate medical plants. The extracts offered include a variety of essential oils, absolutes, plant extracts, macerated oils, tubers, clays, algae, seaweeds and minerals. An animal may choose to inhale what they select, taking it orally, or by it being rubbed on parts of its body.

Over the years, we tried to support Hagrid's health with an array of natural solutions, complemented by veterinary medicine. Usually, for us medications were a last resort. Fortunately, my vet, Graham erred on the side of caution when it came to prescribing antibiotics and steroids for Hagrid, which mirrored my own reluctance to use them. Occasionally however, there were times when I did have to use strong pharmaceutical drugs. Before using them, however, I would research the side effects of the drug in relation to the state of Hagrid's current health.

Then I might delay using them if I felt that the side effects would do more damage than good, especially with the consideration that Hagrid already had a compromised immune system. I always tried to find a natural solution that suited Hagrid.

Before meeting Hagrid, I'd been on a journey learning about my own health, nutrition and digestion. Because of this, I was able to help him by applying a few of the principles I'd learnt.

I wanted to build up his immune system. Zoopharmacognosy can work to support veterinary medicine and help a dog deal better with any side effects medication may cause. Hagrid's early life had involved significant distress and several visits to the vet, plus he'd encountered a number of powerful drugs. It also seemed clear to me that he was having digestive problems, which may have been side effects. I was increasingly confident that he needed to avoid these drugs as much as possible.

Dogs know what their bodies need. If a dog is lacking something in their diet, say iron, they will be drawn towards things that have iron in, as their body is trying to compensate for the lack of it.

Before knowing about self-selection, I'd used canine probiotics in Hagrid's food when he was on any strong pharmaceuticals. And I made that decision because they'd helped me at the time, because while antibiotics will reduce unwanted bacteria, they will also do the same to positive digestive bacteria. The probiotics are good for strengthening the body's restoration while the antibiotics are at work. These were given during the course of antibiotics, and for a few weeks after they had finished.

Later, as I became aware of self-selection, Hagrid had the opportunity to select what would help him. I didn't wait until Hagrid was ill, before giving him the chance to choose from an array of herbs and oils. Under specialist advice, zoopharmacognosy was adapted and continued during medication.

Over time, Hagrid's digestion was dramatically improved and his body became able to absorb nutrients efficiently. In the last four years of his life, there was no more diarrhoea and sickness, which was quite astonishing given where we'd started. I thought that if we could improve Hagrid's health from the inside, what showed on the outside would improve too, so we also worked on his food. He was a dog who would come and ask for certain foods in a subtle way. I listened to what

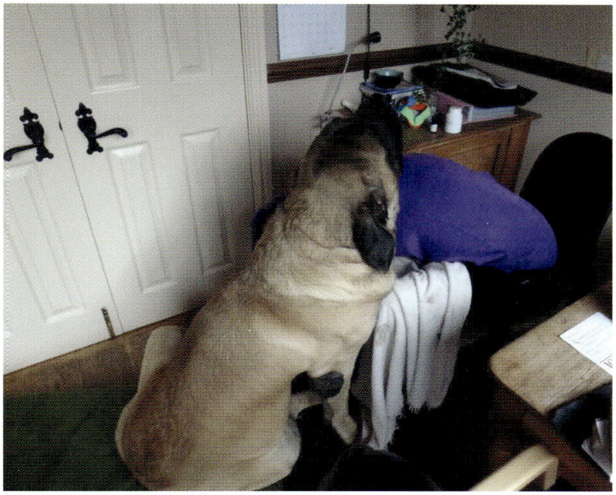

Hagrid comes over and waits for green clay to be put onto his leg.

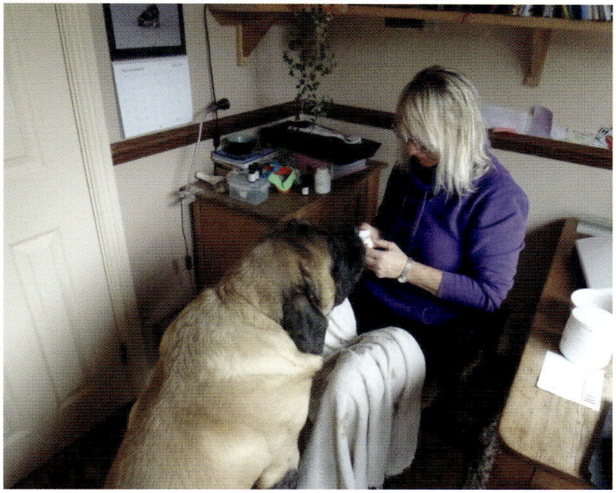

Hagrid sniffing the green clay and oils he'd selected.

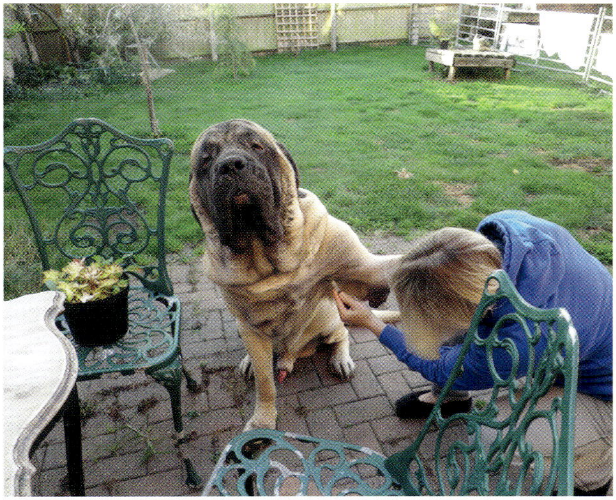

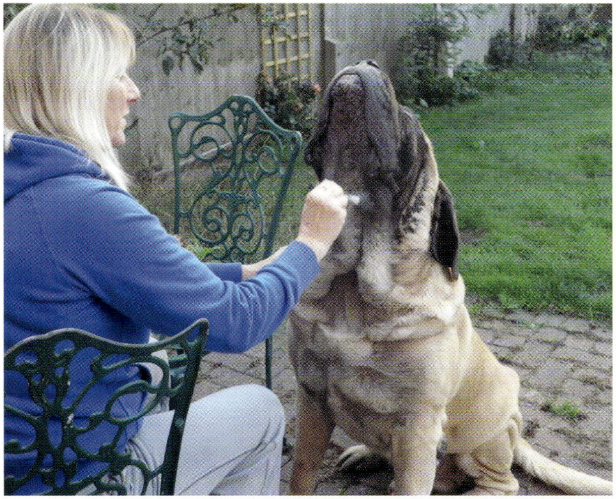

As you can see from these photos, Hagrid enjoyed having the green clay put on his neck. It must have been soothing. He positioned himself like this, his head tilting backwards, which showed me how much he enjoyed it. He has such soft body language; his ears are long and relaxed, his tail is out to the side and his head and jaw are relaxed. Without being trained, Hagrid relished these times by positioning himself when I was preparing for a session.

he was saying and gave them to him. He knew what he needed. These foods were in their natural state, unprocessed, without additives, colourings, salt or anything poisonous to dogs. There were vegetables and fruits such as bananas, carrots, eggs, coconut; foods recognisable in their natural form.

When one of our dogs tells us he's interested in a certain food, we're guided by his choice, if it's appropriate. This is different from us deciding and supplementing their diet with what we think may benefit them. Because Hagrid had allergies, we were careful, so just one or two foods could be added at a time with weeks in between.

Self-selection as prevention and health care is relatively new for dogs and other animals. As far as I'm aware at the time of writing, self-selecting safe, appropriate food is virtually unknown in the dog world. Perhaps it's something to be explored as a holistic way forward. Obviously the dog needs to be in a position of feeling calm and secure – to be able to make sensible decisions.

A deeper look at self-selection

Self-selection gives any animal, people included, a rare opportunity to heal themselves, whether or not any medical condition has been diagnosed. It's often used as preventative medicine and may also be referred to as wild health, because wild animals have been documented to select herbs, grasses, and minerals from their environment. They choose various plant extracts at different times of the year to meet their specific needs and some know where to go for it. This knowledge is innate in all animals.

In the wild, before domestication and urbanisation, animals would have had a wide selection of plants and substances to choose from. Now they're domestic, these choices are much more limited to them. Their lifestyles have changed dramatically, and so has the human-controlled environment in which they live. Dogs have little choice about most things in their lives. Animals will try to seek out what they can from what's available, even if the options are limited. And through self-selection, we can enlarge that selection so they can help keep themselves balanced.

It's not uncommon for dogs to eat plant material other than grass, such as bark, berries, shrubs, chalk, earth and so on. This is just one example of them knowing how to help themselves when they need it.

A dog may chew at an unusual material because there is an ingredient contained within it that they need. There are reasons for dogs eating grass and faeces, for example. My dogs will eat it now and then and I feel for them this isn't a problem, although it may be for some dogs. At other times they may eat much more than usual and I've noted at times they can be under pressure of some description. Because of certain factors in their lives or diet, they may actually need something that's in the unnatural food, indicating that they're out of balance at that time.

Giving dogs a choice of safe, appropriate materials they wouldn't otherwise have, helps them to keep themselves well. Believe it or not, they often instinctively know more about themselves than some might think. It's interesting to see, and I see it a lot, that once an animal's needs have been met with zoopharmacognosy, it's less likely they will look for other options.

Self-selection for Hagrid

I don't think that Hagrid would have reached eight and a half years of age without self-selection. The changes in him were so clear. He chose certain things, like Green Clay, Spirulina and Aloe Vera, and wanted to have them frequently. Sometimes he'd change his preferences, but because he had access to self-selection on a regular basis, this seemed to give him a solid base, and his immune system became much stronger. In fact, he became stronger in every way. His behaviour improved and he tolerated people much better. He grew healthier as he aged, which I found quite amazing. Once his base health became established, several of his other complaints disappeared and he was able to tolerate much more in the way of foods.

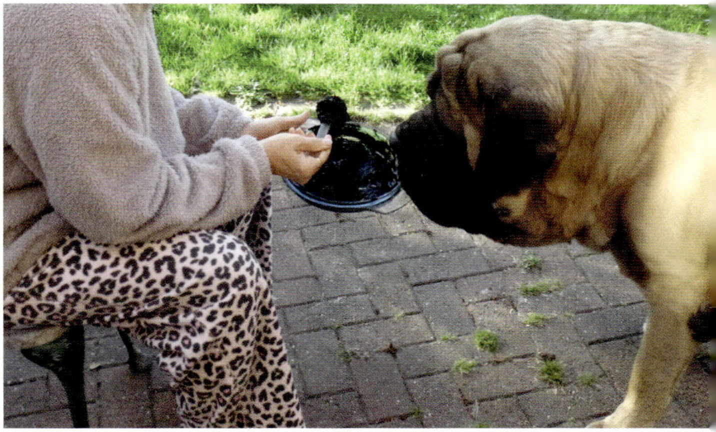

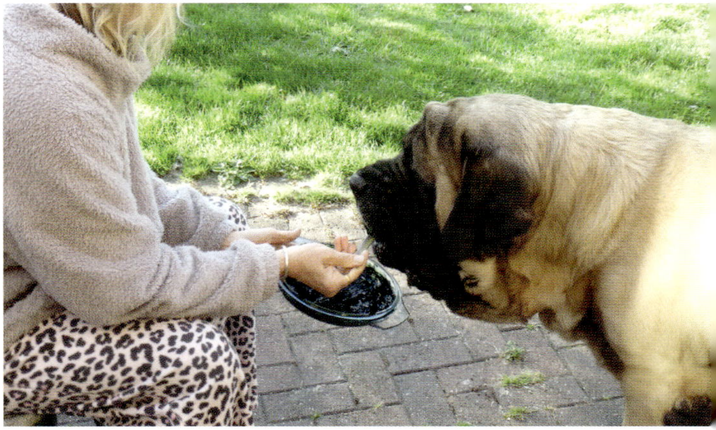

Hagrid loved to have very thick spirulina most days. My other dogs prefer spirulina quite watered down Although he managed to eat some by himself, he found it easier this way. He was usually very green afterwards! We did this outside because it's terribly messy! Towels were very useful too.

Zoopharmacognosy can also be used for more targeted situation-based help, as we did a couple of times when Hagrid had infections in a wound on his leg. He selected oils and in time the infection cleared up, saving him the difficulty of a trip to the vet and antibiotics. Not only could he build resistance against them, but now there's quite a lot of evidence to say that using antibiotics can be detrimental to the immune system, especially when used too much.

We wanted to avoid using medication whenever we could; saving them for times when it really was necessary. This meant we'd monitor him daily, offering zoopharmacognosy, feeding a quality diet as much as possible and trying to limit distress with the lifestyle choices we made.

Maybe Hagrid – just like some lifelong human sufferers of chronic poor health – adopted a different, perhaps even brighter outlook on life. He seemed contented and comfortable with a slower way of being. This meant going out for walks almost every day, in a variety of areas, chosen for his needs and skills at the time. He'd have a walk, sit and view his surroundings, occasionally walk with a familiar known dog, with tracking included every so often.

This was Hagrid's world, and he really did come to embody the 'less is more' approach to life.

Chapter 16

Food

In 2007 while on a short break, I started to read a book called *The Allergy Connection* by Barbara Paterson. It made total sense to me and I instinctively related to what I was reading. On coming home I immediately stopped eating sugar, dairy and wheat. At the same time, I gradually began taking myself off anti-depressants (Venlafaxine) and quit smoking.

Perhaps I did too much at once, and there were side effects, but I stuck to it because after a week I was reluctant to go back to any of them, despite being quite ill. It had taken a lot of energy to last a week. In hindsight, doing one thing at a time might have been better. But the book woke me up, and facing reality without all the crutches was quite revealing and I couldn't bear to be poisoning my body a moment longer, which was how it felt at the time. I learnt to have emotions again, and life was raw for some time while I worked through all of this.

Next, a nutritionist helped guide me through the maze of what was okay for me and what wasn't. Fiona, the person who guides me now and has done for several years is mentioned at the end of the chapter. Now and then there are tests that I take, and Fiona translates the results, considers other elements in my life and makes suggestions with food choices and supplements. Later I give her feedback to see if any more changes are needed.

Nowadays, I'm much more aware of the way my body works and what effects some foods have. It's quite surprising how certain foods can change my mood dramatically and the other impacts some may have. We all know the effects that alcohol has on most people's frame of mind and it affects everyone in various ways; some know when to stop and others carry on. The same principle applies to food. Over time, since improving my diet and digestion, the symptoms of Irritable Bowel Syndrome I used to have significantly improved, and it's not an issue these days.

The impact of food on mood applies to dogs too. They're also affected by what they eat, how regular the food is, what's happening in their lives and how their digestion works as a result. The dogs who live with us now have four meals of quality food every day. Some of these meals they choose, within limits, and I'm sure we could go further with the idea of self-selection for meals, in time. All the dogs we share our lives with have come from previous homes, and each has typically brought some kind of issue with them, for example, they're 'unwanted'. This can mean that they've experienced a breakdown in relationships, and so already they're at an emotional, and by implication physical, disadvantage.

Looking directly at their carer is one way that dogs communicate. This may be when they need to go out to the toilet, go for a walk, would like some attention, guidance, they're hungry, or for something else. It could simply be because they like their carer and are happy being with them. When we love someone, we often like to look with softness, just gazing at them. Dogs do that too, and I'm sure for the same kind of reasons. There are those questioning looks, appreciative ones too. Dogs have ways of saying they are grateful, satisfied, fulfilled and happy about something with just a look. There are also looks when they're sad because something bad has happened, or unhappy because of feeling unwell. Some are because they're scared, anxious, uncertain or want to avoid something and those may be accompanied by showing the whites of their eye (whale eye). Then there are expressions of disgust and dissatisfaction. As you can imagine, dogs give looks for a variety of reasons.

There was a look my dogs used to give when they wanted food or treats. They would also give me a different look if I moved in a particular way that may have meant something was about to happen, or they picked up on what I was thinking at that time in the day. Occasionally I would wonder if they could read my mind, as they seemed to at times. Although we may not think so, we're actually quite predictable, and dogs, among other animals, learn to pick up on our patterns.

I found that by not giving treats for behaviour, the urgency and expectation wasn't there and the dogs were calmer and more carefree. For some of them it took time to adapt to the change, depending on their background and experiences. Also, leaving treats out of our lives has allowed for a much more relaxed feel to the relationship. The dogs can ask for what they want, I can listen and give them that if it's applicable at the time. We have a much more honest relationship because food isn't being used as a reward or coercion for something they've done or that I'd like them to do.

To begin with, Hagrid was fed the same commercial diet he'd been given in his previous home, but it offered him little in the way of nutritional benefit. In his first few weeks with us, there had been so many changes for him that I wasn't going to switch his diet so soon. In that initial settling-in period, I would have preferred to maintain consistency in his diet for longer, at least for the first few weeks. However, it was evident from day one that there was a problem, and while I'd expected some initial upset from a dog that's been re-homed, he soon had fairly bad diarrhoea.

Twice in his life Hagrid was on kibble-type prescription diets. One seemed to keep symptoms at bay, but the manufacturer changed the source of protein, and soon afterwards we discovered that the new one didn't suit him. The times he was on commercial diets, I noticed that he was really keen to eat vegetables, which Hagrid asked me for, and eventually I gave in to this as other symptoms developed. I say 'give in to this' because when feeding a dog who has allergies, they are meant to have the same food, otherwise how is it possible to trace what has caused a flare up?

I noticed a direct link to a worsening in his conditions each time he was on a course of antibiotic and anti-inflammatories. New sores popped up, his feet would become swollen, and his diarrhoea invariably re-occurred. We stuck with the home-prepared diet, which was relatively basic, and gradually it worked.

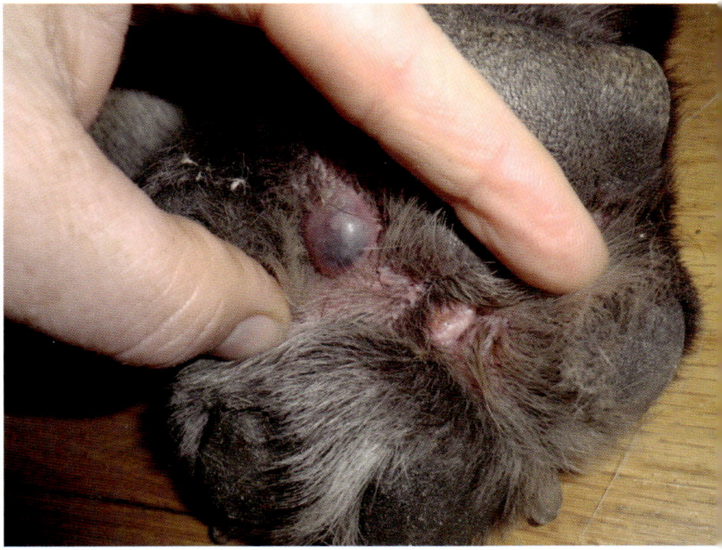

This would happen at the time or after antibiotics were used.

Often, we'd find that some kind of food suited Hagrid, and we'd continue with it for quite some time, but he would eventually become sensitive to it. Over the months I started to bring new sources of protein into his diet - slowly, not wanting to cause any upset, and observed his response.

Hagrid was fed three times a day, as was normal for our other dogs at the time. Having regular meals, little and often, keeps dogs sustained and fulfilled, which impacts positively on their behaviour; it keeps them more balanced. I've found that this limits, or even stops, their need to steal food. They feel satisfied, and when out and about they'll often resist the temptation to wolf down anything they can find.

Some time ago, a dog came to stay with us who was used to being fed one meal of commercial biscuits a day. He showed anxious behaviour while the food was being prepared and gulped it down. As the other dogs who lived with me were fed three times a day, it seemed only fair to do the same for him, so I divided up his daily allowance. By the second day of this routine, he'd begun to leave a few of his biscuits and was less animated while food was being prepared.

A dog who is fed several meals a day is likely to be able to communicate his preferences by leaving bits he doesn't like. A dog fed once a day who doesn't like the food is probably going to eat it because it's all there is, whether suitable or not.

I'm sure that if I were fed once a day I'd bolt down the food, knowing that the next time I'd have food would be twenty-four hours later! I've actually tried this a few times and my main focus really was on food. I became irritable, found it hard to concentrate on much else nearer the time of a meal and then when it came, I enjoyed it but ate more quickly and wanted more. Afterwards I had indigestion and stomach pains. If this was done every day, it would soon become a big concern in my life, and any delay would certainly lead to significant anxiety. Also remember that we control this aspect of a dog's life entirely, and I believe that it's because having such little control over food that some problems arise for a few.

It's nice when a dog's able to express their concerns if they're unhappy with what they're eating. I imagine people would like the same choices. When I'm hungry, I'm definitely more wired, on edge and likely to be more irritable. In comparison, if I've just eaten, I can relax, reflect *and* sleep better.

At one point, Hagrid was having five small meals a day to aid his digestion. His food was served in crockery mixing bowls, this is because plastic seeps into food or water and the dogs preferred ceramic bowls for water. Christopher Day, the homeopathic vet, had first suggested we check the material used for the dogs' bowls as Hagrid had allergies and this could affect them. Due to his allergies, choosing a home-prepared diet seemed the most sensible option, so that we could eliminate certain foods to check whether he was sensitive to them. This was difficult at the beginning and it didn't help that he had several necessary courses of antibiotics and anti-inflammatories as well.

It was challenging to feed Hagrid because his sensitivities kept changing and over the years we tried several different diets. Amongst these was a raw food diet, which worked well for a while. I'll add here that, although I've heard that in many circumstances raw food can help clear up skin conditions 'like magic', for Hagrid it helped short-term, but not for very long. Nothing did. I tried to keep the variety going with the raw food but it really didn't provide the solution for us.

To begin with, most diets seemed to help Hagrid, but none of them made all of his symptoms clear up completely and some improvements lasted longer than others. Certain products and food combinations felt right, but others most definitely didn't. I remember that one of the commercial diets he only ate reluctantly, and it happened to be one that didn't feel right to me either.

Feeding him something the vet had recommended, but I knew he wasn't enjoying, was very hard to do. We used the recommended dried biscuits and tinned foods, both on prescription, to add some variety, and regularly gave meals in a Kong. This was to keep his interest as he was unable to have bones, treats and so on. At times, on commercial dried prescription diets, Hagrid's ears oozed brown fluid, which was different from when on a home-prepared or raw diet. These diets always had the same effect; he drank much more (despite the food being soaked in water). He'd even regularly wake us in the night to go out to eat grass. Hagrid seemed focused almost to the point of obsession about eating grass, he was desperate for something and regularly ate from the compost heap, too.

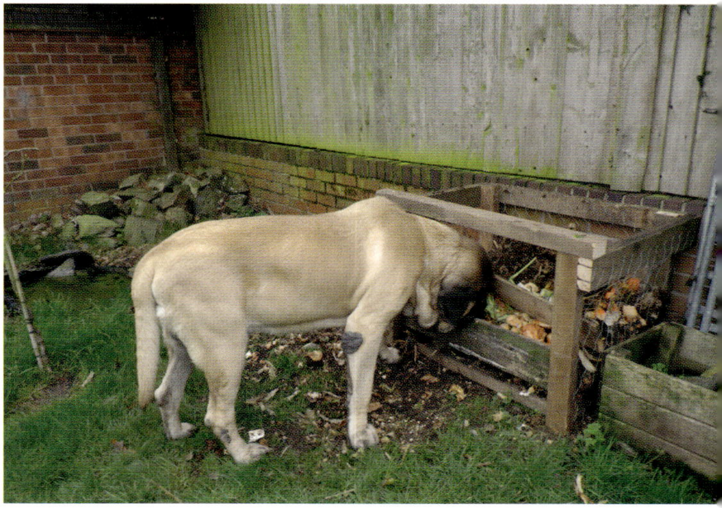

The compost heap where Hagrid desperately sought out vegetable matter when on a prescription diet.

Some of the diets I tried for Hagrid

- Sweet potato, lamb, lentils and chicken (alternating the meat along with a limited variety of vegetables).
- Cooked rabbit (which he chose) and cooked sweet potato.
- Cooked kangaroo, bought in bulk, which turned out not to suit him at all.
- Different types of cooked fish in rotation, with a variety of raw vegetables; this sustained him for over a year and he really enjoyed sprats, mackerel, salmon, coley and pollock (a kind local butcher, Bill Spencer, sourced the fish for Hagrid and went out of his way to find various suppliers of what we'd asked for).
- Raw commercial diet, although only one variety suited him.
- Lentils and vegetables rotated with fish.
- Chickpeas (these caused wind, and having wind regularly is a sign that something in the diet may not be suiting a dog).
- Quinoa, nuts and eggs (please note that some nuts are poisonous for dogs).
- Raw rabbit and vegetables.

In a local field, on several occasions, Hagrid dug down a little way into the soil and ate small amounts of earth, staying there for ten to fifteen minutes. He obviously needed to do this and knew exactly where to go and what to do. He acted with determination and a sense of purpose. It was clearly necessary for him and I thought he was clever because he only ever used this behaviour in that particular field, which hadn't been used for years, so hadn't any herbicides or pesticides on it.

Some people might stop dogs from eating certain plants and soil; although there are some which are unsafe for dogs, it's worth checking first and becoming familiar with what may be toxic.

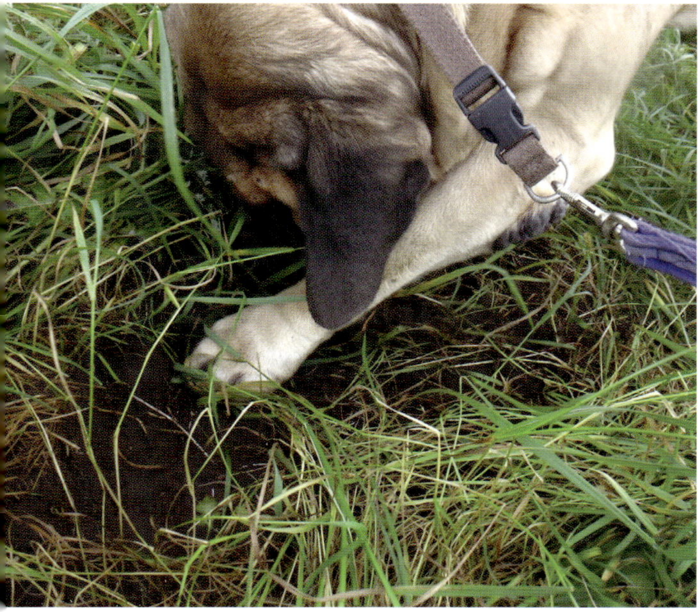

If a dog's eating particular plants, they probably need something from them and we can try to find out what they require. Further investigation, possibly via zoopharmacognosy, could enable them to find what they need. Please see the chapter on zoopharmacognosy for more information.

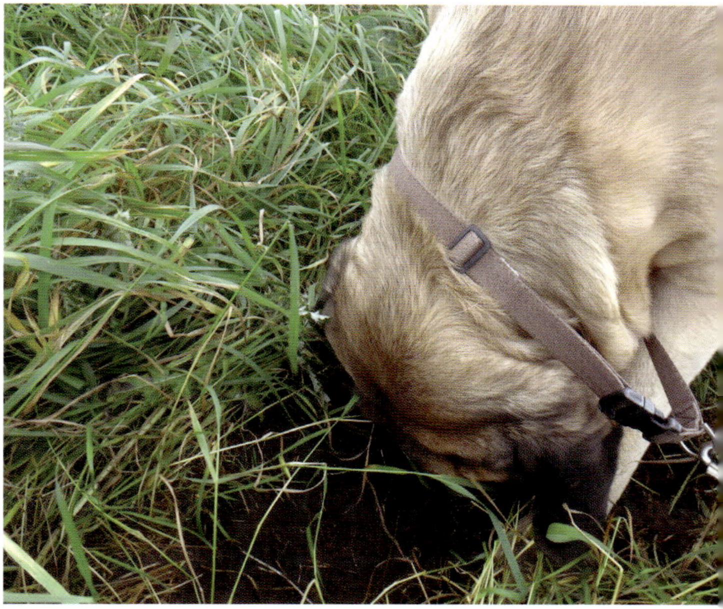

Here, Hagrid is digging and inhaling the soil in a field that had been left fallow for years. He knew what he needed and went in search of it; I followed.

In the past, Henry our Clumber Spaniel was limited to a diet of chicken and potato because of having Inflammatory Bowel Disease (IBD), which had been caused mostly by lifestyle. At that time Henry would come running with me, which I thought was beneficial for him, not recognising that he didn't really have a choice, as most dogs who do these activities don't.

I was a pet-sitter and invariably clients' dogs would stay with us. This frequently interrupted Henry's routine. On top of these factors, which I hadn't realised contributed to his IBD, we'd been asked to ensure that he was kept muzzled, to stop him eating things that the vet didn't allow.

Despite this and being walked on-lead, he still managed to get other food through his muzzle. The distress caused by stopping him from eating what he really wanted (and probably needed), I'm sure was far worse than the cure. He had a terrible life made worse by these restrictions and died aged just six years old.

I felt so sorry for Henry and was aware of his unhappiness so I took his muzzle off when he went to sleep, and sometimes on walks because he was on-lead, depending on where we were. He was always eager to eat grass and having a muzzled dog is something I really struggle with when it's evident the dog is unhappy, depressed and distressed by it, as Henry so obviously was. If a dog does have to wear a muzzle for legal reasons it's important they have time to get used to it and it's comfortable.

For Hagrid, I'd moved on and wasn't prepared to stick with something that was causing him distress. With him, I was always weighing up what was happening in all aspects of his mental and physical condition and making appropriate decisions.

Detecting the source of issues

Finding the cause of particular symptoms was difficult. Some foods were obvious culprits, so we avoided them and only tried them again much later. Although there were gradual improvements over the years, finding totally suitable foods was almost impossible. When we discovered self-selection recommended by Sheila Harper and Winny Boerman, Hagrid regularly selected spirulina and green clay and, with time and consistency, I feel there was quite a significant improvement in his digestion and health overall. That was evident just by looking at him and his faeces. He was able to consume a greater variety of foods with not so many ill effects.

Other changes we made were also factors that could have contributed to his wellness. While it was possible to see direct correlations with flare ups and

Hagrid's condition, sometimes I really struggled to find a definitive answer: I was never sure whether it was his food, environment, emotional state, or a combination of a few of them, that had altered the equilibrium of his health.

Despite not always knowing what triggered a flare-up of one of his conditions, one thing I went along with was Hagrid's ability to communicate his choice of foods. I was fascinated to see him select raw carrot, coconut, raw and cooked beetroot, radishes, bananas, grapefruit, blackberries, watermelon, eggs along with shells from crabs and other things. He didn't show interest in all the food I prepared, he was selective.

When I'm in the kitchen and dealing with food, there are often bits and pieces the dogs show interest in, then I offer them small pieces of cauliflower, carrot, coconut and chicken, for example. This may not be every day but the dogs can watch and sometimes choose to be in the kitchen. Usually, the smell of a particular food will bring them in, and this is how Hagrid told me what he needed. He'd show me by standing close and resting his head on the work surface if I hadn't got the message. I listened to him because I could tell how strongly he required the food. He didn't always appear when I was getting meals ready, he just came when I would be preparing and cooking particular food. Sometimes he'd be a little interested, and at other times he'd seem like he really wanted whatever it was.

To me, his level of interest was in a way a reflection of how much he needed it in his diet at the time. The example from earlier, about how he had to eat grass so much when he was on a limited diet that he'd wake us up at night to go out, is a good way of showing what I mean. His body really craved it because the diet was so lacking, and that was reflected in how strongly he tried to communicate his intention.

When a dog comes to live with us, they often come with the idea that food is the most important thing in the world. Most of them appeared to be ravenous, stealing and eating the wrapper the food came in, raiding bins and guarding food. And it's possible for a dog to have issues with absorbing some foods.

Hagrid was pretty keen on food, but he wasn't the keenest dog I've come across; distress can be a reason for this sort of orientation, as well as an inappropriate diet that doesn't sustain them. For some dogs new to a home, this would be a significant point of change, and therefore it creates some obvious unease. Equally, on the reverse side of things, others can lose their appetite during these times.

We've realised giving several meals a day works best, up to four or five depending on the dog's needs. Each one is fed alone, with a physical barrier between them and any other animals. Many like privacy when eating and can eat at their own pace. Some are affected by another dog checking their bowl after they've finished, so I pick the bowls up when they have eaten. It's possible that a few can have pre-existing sensitivities around food from living with other dogs, so if these things are done, it helps them to feel at ease.

Occasionally my dogs like things to chew after their meal. It doesn't have to be food (they could be wooden chews for example), as long as they're safe and are given to them individually so that they don't feel another dog will take them. Some dogs will require physical boundaries. Pogo had a tough past and needs to know that what she is given is hers. Even though she's better now, there are times when she still needs these boundaries.

I also give my dogs meals in different ways now and then to make things more interesting. This could be small pieces of food wrapped in paper then put in a cardboard box; or an empty milk carton with holes cut out and stuffed with kitchen roll. I need to point out that these items are safe for my dogs but may not be for every dog. Sometimes they can be fed in different places in the house or the garden. I might do this every so often as it makes things more involving for them while always monitoring their level of excitement.

Not all dogs are comfortable eating in a different place at first; it can make them feel vulnerable. If any of mine are out in the garden, I stay around because they may need support to feel safe. In my experience, quite a few dogs feel vulnerable out in the garden on their own and it's often a reason for them barking or coming in and toileting indoors. They're quite simply worried in some way.

The properties of different foods

When I researched the properties of the foods Hagrid was selecting, it amazed me. A few of them are shown opposite.

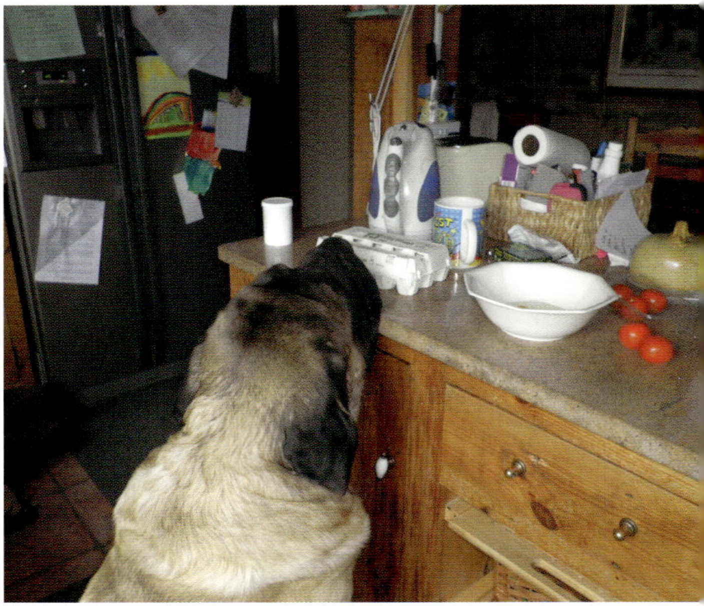

Hagrid asks for raw eggs.

Carrots

These are antioxidant, anti-inflammatory, useful for remedying cognitive dysfunction and may help restore vision with beta-carotene.

Coconut

The dogs and I regularly shared a coconut. I read later how beneficial they are. Coconut improves digestion, is an anti-inflammatory, helps promote healthy thyroid, and gives the body energy. It's anti-fungal, antiviral, anti-parasitic, anti-bacterial, improves the immune system, is good for the heart and so much more! Isn't that amazing? Both Pogo and Hagrid showed real interest in them.

Bananas

As well as being an anti-inflammatory and containing vitamin C, bananas are also considered a tonic for the brain because of two substances found within them; tryptophan and magnesium, which together help the body produce serotonin. Bananas also have a high potassium ratio, helping to lower blood pressure and boost alertness. These were another favourite Hagrid often selected, but only when he needed them. Despite being a huge dog, two or three were usually enough for him; intermittently, not as a daily supplement.

Beetroot

This is used for skin problems, is an anti-oxidant, and contains nitrates that promote the flow of blood and take oxygen to places where it's lacking. It also increases the number of white blood cells used for fighting infection and diseases, and contains Glutamine, which is an amino acid for maintaining the intestinal tract.

Eggs

Eggs build the immune system, contain Choline (important for the brain), are good for the health of eyes, contain Omega 3 fats, are a good source of protein and fat, and aid the thyroid gland.

Grapefruit

High in vitamin C, contains Lycopene (found in the pink and red varieties) and has anti-tumour properties. This was very interesting because he definitely showed a strong interest in it when I ate grapefruit in the evenings. As soon as I had some, he'd be there, but when I offered it to him, although he was very keen, he didn't take any. It was obvious he wanted some, but how? That's when it was suggested that I offered grapefruit essential oil mixed with aloe vera gel and some water.

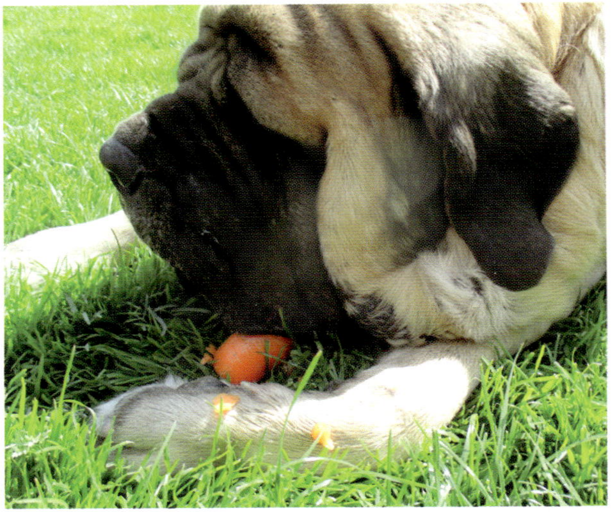

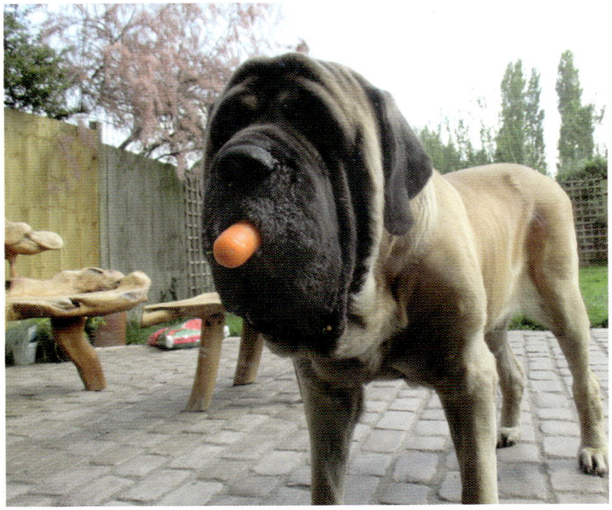

Hagrid eating carrots outside. Sometimes he'd get up and come to the door to be let in and eat it in his bed.

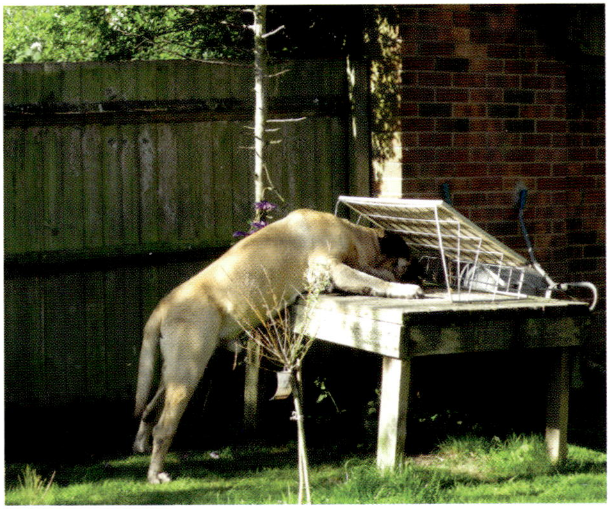

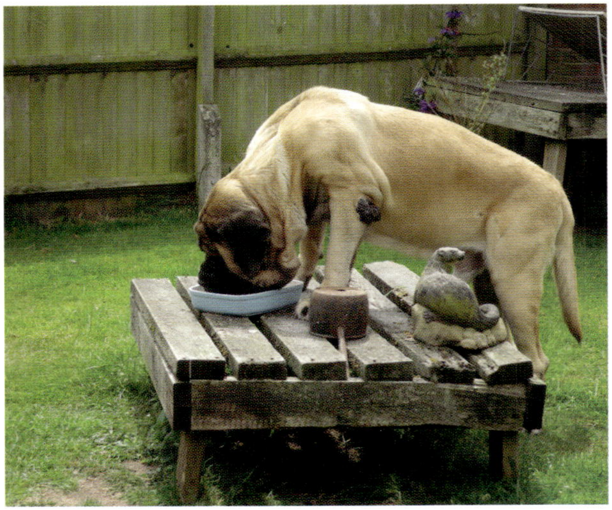

What's this on our bird table?

Allowing exploration

Hagrid's communication was always extremely difficult to read, even for people who were exceptionally experienced. I wonder how much of that lying low that he learned early on in his life came into play. He really was so sensitive and easily put off if he felt any kind of pressure or threat. To a large extent, I was able to read him and I experienced instinctive feelings of him wanting something or not, so I went with that. Near the end of his life, I definitely felt he didn't want any more oils and I could no longer tell, so for the last few days he didn't have them. I just hope that I got it right for him.

Because our animals have choices, it was fine if Hagrid chose to eat from the bird table. Asking him to get off was something I could have done quite calmly and nicely, and he would have done what I asked. But I use requests sparingly because it's easy to nag a dog when they do things we don't want them to. A brief moment to decide whether things are acceptable is all that's required, and if it's something that isn't, it's usually possible to change at a later point. There's never been a life-threatening situation or anything that's called for more than a polite request.

Hagrid made the decision to check out the bird table and as he'd been unable to make many choices in his previous life, because of being bullied, I wanted to encourage his self-esteem. If I'd wanted to stop Hagrid from eating from the table, rather than destroy his confidence or make it an issue, I would have left him this one time, then put something around it to stop him from getting to it. This kind of physical prevention doesn't have the negative emotional impact that telling him to stop would have.

However, if I did need him to come away from it right then, distracting him with something would work. Going into the garage or getting on with some gardening would be enough, because he'd want to come and see what I was doing. Another option would be to feed the birds in a different manner or place.

It's so easy to quash a sensitive dog's self-confidence by nagging or shouting, impacting on trust and the relationship. For Hagrid to investigate and make other choices showed that he was growing in confidence and this was a chance for me to learn more about him. Rather than intervening, I decided it was a good idea to observe, after all there was no harm being done.

At one time I might have rushed in, panicking; now I've learnt that such a response can take away confidence. He had worked out what to do to get to the food there and needed it at that time: maybe he just wanted to see if anything was left?

Notes on dietary advice

What constitutes a healthy diet varies between people. I can choose to take advice from a qualified nutritionist and research the information. I can make informed decisions and adjustments to my diet and monitor any differences these changes make. In the dog world, this approach to nutrition is a relatively new field.

As far as I'm aware at the time of writing, there are no equivalent standards for a canine nutritionist, so seeking out good quality professional support is a real challenge. I hope now that we're moving on.

However, we can look out for pointers ourselves to explore whether certain foods are suitable for our dogs. These include observing the quality of their coat, skin, faeces, teeth, eyes, behaviour and sleep.

I use the guidelines opposite as a measure, though in my experience they are suitable for most dogs.

The long-term effect of feeding one food only is taken into account and I always offer a varied diet – many of us humans have this for the obvious health benefits it provides and I proceed with caution.

At the end of this chapter are book ideas and contact details of people who can provide more specialised support and advice in this area.

- I've found it's best to avoid additives including salt and sugar.
- There are foods that could be poisonous to dogs. I research foods of which I'm unsure. A few are macadamia nuts, chocolate, coffee, xylitol, some fruits, but there are others that can be found online.
- My dogs have some say in their diet. If the dog in question is one who eats anything and everything, then other areas of their life may need looking at before they're able to genuinely let me know what they prefer. You will have read that some foods were detrimental to Hagrid's health. This can apply to any dog.
- I find foods that are fulfilling for my dogs, and consider the number of meals each individual requires.

Why it is important to take guidance on diet

Although food can be a large contributor to good or bad health, there are many other factors that come into it at the same time. These include:

- lifestyle, environment, exercise, health, age, sleep and rest
- living with other dogs/animals
- the dog's perspective of the relationship with the carer and other family members
- contentment, and maybe loneliness, or in some cases boredom

All of the above can impact on how the dog's digestive system will work and therefore their food requirements. Nowadays I consider the whole landscape of a dog's life when looking at causes and choices.

I've decided to include a few suggestions of books that helped me with my health and diet. Having been involved with a nutritionist for a few years and learning about the importance of human nutrition, I began asking questions about what would be helpful for my dogs. So having a foundation of understanding in human nutrition, it's easy to see how food impacts on our lives, and so in our dogs' lives.

A great resource is Robert Sapolsky's stress lectures (see the *Further reading* chapter at the end of the book). Although he focuses on the human response to stress, it can translate well to dogs. A book I read quite early on, which was an excellent guide and an informative read, was Gut and Psychology Syndrome by Dr. Natasha Campbell-McBride. Also, look out for human nutritionist Fiona Mealing from Suffolk who has a lot of useful information about what we put into our bodies.

Other great books include:

From Stress to Success
by Xandria Williams.

Hidden Food Allergies
by Patrick Holford.

Food is Better Medicine than Drugs
by Patrick Holford.

Too Young to Grow Old
by Anne-Lise Miller.

Wild Health
by Cindy Engel.

Key points

- In Hagrid's first few weeks with us, there were so many changes for him that I decided not to switch his diet too soon.
- I noticed a direct link to a worsening in his conditions each time he was on a course of antibiotic and anti-inflammatories.
- Having regular meals, little and often, keeps my dogs sustained and fulfilled, which impacts positively on their behaviour; it keeps them more balanced.
- What I've found is that a dog who is fed several meals a day is likely to be able to communicate his preferences by leaving bits he doesn't like.
- I was a pet-sitter and invariably clients' dogs would stay with us. This can interrupt dogs' routine.
- Many dogs like privacy when eating and can then eat at their own pace. Some are affected by another dog checking their bowl after they've finished, so I pick up their bowls later, when they have eaten.
- Hagrid made the decision to check out the bird table. As he'd been unable to make many decisions in his previous life because of being bullied, I allowed him to investigate as I wanted to encourage his self-esteem and decision-making.

Chapter 17

Innate dexterity

I'm often intrigued by my dogs' ability to self-regulate and make their own decisions. It's within them, as part of their natural makeup. I believe this intuition spans all aspects of their lives; physical movement, diet, relationships, emotional needs, and overall decision-making. As dogs have this capability for balance in them already, the best way to approach improving their lives, without changing anything else, is to work together to guide them to a place where they can co-ordinate their behaviour themselves, and let *that* lead our work with them.

This is perhaps a shift in thinking; from seeing a dog as a set of behavioural issues to be solved one by one, to trying to build them up using their own natural regulation of thoughts and feelings as a basis, and then to develop from there. Most of us choose to live like this in our own lives every day. It's an amazing freedom we have to be able to make our own decisions, and live our own lives, because we know what we want and what's best for us. And I think dogs do too, even though culturally there's a belief that they don't. Humans make mistakes every day and hopefully learn from them. Could dogs be offered a similar opportunity?

Because dogs live in *our* world, which is largely alien to them and caters towards humans and what we innately understand, this natural sense of self-regulation often gets confused. In short, dogs don't understand or even fit in with a lot of the world that they live in; they're our guests, but they don't really belong here. For some, this can lead to confusion and strange (to humans) behaviour, to the point that it might seem that they don't know what they're doing or know what's best for them.

If a dog is coming from a good place mentally, has support and guidance, everything else is likely to follow. And the first step in helping them reach this point is to recognise what is needed. This is why I have given it a name; innate dexterity, and why I've devoted a chapter to defining and exploring it. For both human and dog, progress begins with observation and understanding.

From my experience over the years and work in understanding dogs, their communication and behaviour, I've found that they are more than capable of making balanced decisions. Then they can have a life that allows for relaxation, comfort, assurance and to be in situations that they can manage.

I've used the word *innate* because what I want to describe is something that each dog is born with. I've found it happens mainly in a natural setting, for example on a walk, although it can be anywhere provided the dog has a settled environment, one where he feels totally relaxed. Coming from a place of thinking clearly, they're in a position to use their brain and body in unison. I liken it to meditation for dogs, and for the handler. Once the dog is in the right frame of mind, they can select movements that are influenced solely by them, within safe limitations, which is where carers come in.

The word *dexterity* was chosen because the dog uses the skill of thinking to move without risk. I believe this is how my dogs' quality of life can be preserved. On any walk, dogs are faced with stimuli and choices of what to do. When thinking clearly he has more chance of making positive decisions and learning how best to use his brain and body in various scenarios. This was something I loved about walks with Hagrid. My dogs and I share this activity and are both using our brains and bodies as we experience life together.

I started with them on-lead. On each dog's individual walk I need to put in appropriate and reasonable limits on their line (long lead) for the particular one I'm with, so that together we experience and enjoy a flowing exploratory walk.

A dog might choose to jump onto a log, stretch into bushes, or be inquisitive to investigate a hole, and all this is safe and possible, supported by the lead.

I'd like to share a walk that Pogo and I had:

As we were navigating our way through a field, I became aware of how skilled Pogo was at making life easier for the sheep by using her body to deflect attention away from them. Maybe she was taking care of the sheep here, and maybe she was keeping herself safe. While she didn't appear on the surface to be particularly worried, there were more of them than there were of her, and they're much bigger! A thinking dog will do what they need to keep themselves safe. In this case Pogo was showing body awareness, which meant she was slowly ambling and in the right frame of mind for innate dexterity. She was thinking clearly and making sensible choices. Another dog might have seen the sheep, been over-excited by them, run over and gotten into a difficult situation because they weren't thinking properly.

Some dogs, like some humans, have the ability to take care of others, whether those they are caring for are other dogs, animals or humans. Pogo does this, and to take some responsibility from her I am on the lookout for times to take that pressure off. One way is to use the lead accordingly and together we made a slow, spacious curve around the sheep, to give them as much room as possible. That's what we did.

In addition to curving her body, Pogo slowed down, sniffed, and generally kept her head low and turned away from them. She moved slowly so she didn't make direct eye contact too. At the same time, to mirror her body language and help her with what she was trying to do, I fleetingly gazed toward the sheep, then looked away, to avoid a direct stare which can come across as confrontational.

When the moment is right, we can learn directly from our dogs, about how to deal with these kinds of meetings and how to make our presence more tolerable for others. Part of this is also respecting their communication; as their carer we have a duty of care to help them with these things. So for example, this would be respecting what they're saying when they communicate not wanting to go in a certain direction. My dogs let me know when they'd rather not go to a particular place and often when I think back to the last time we've been in an area, I can remember something happening, some kind of fear; a dog barking from behind a fence, or them meeting an over-excited dog.

Adding into that is the fact that they can smell what's been there before, and we can't. On one particular route, my dogs were able to tell where there was the fresh scent of a particular dog, and would usually avoid going that way. One of them chose to avoid walks in that area altogether. There could be environmental factors or memories of past experiences that may cause any dog to be cautious about a certain place they don't like going to.

Being barked at is similar to us being shouted at, so helping them find alternative routes, if this is the case, can prevent this upset. As a side note, dogs that bark from their gardens or houses usually do it because they're worried about something. They're barking because they feel vulnerable, not because they enjoy it. So avoiding these routes is essentially respecting their space; that is, my own dogs' and the other dogs'. Some may not have many choices in their lives, especially if they're farm animals, so it's also nice to help them.

On this walk, Pogo used sniffing for several reasons: Sometimes it occurred because there was something interesting, at other times she used it as a distraction technique, for example, to look occupied, as we might do with our phones! Sniffing slows dogs down, giving them time, an opportunity for clearer thinking and while this happens they become more aware of their bodies and movements made.

Not only does it slow the sniffing dog down it's a clear message to others that the attention is off them, so giving the other time and space to make a decision. In effect their communication improves when they have more time to think and move slowly, just as we might. This helped Pogo as well as the other animals.

Sniffing can also be used because the dog is worried about their surroundings so will 'over sniff' to block the environment out. I didn't think the sheep worried her; she was okay to be on-lead in a field with them as she investigated. If Pogo was in a field of rabbits though, which for her is more exciting, it might have been different. Or maybe we'd avoid that area altogether as we used to, because it could be too intense. Then there's always the option of turning around and going back; these are some choices and decisions we have available that would help a dog remain in a settled frame of mind, to get the most out of their walk.

These days, and because of the work we've done together over the years, Pogo is able to come down quickly after being excited by seeing rabbits running, though that hadn't always been the case!

All Pogo and I aim to do is have a calm time on our walk, and we work together to achieve this.

Once we were out of the field of sheep, I unclipped her lead gently and we pottered along the lane a little way. Pogo stayed fairly close, checking in with me now and then as we were walking. Then I noticed she caught the smell of something; the scent was interesting and took her up the steep bank where she continued exploring a rabbit burrow for quite a while, staying longer than she usually would around the burrows. It looked like another animal had

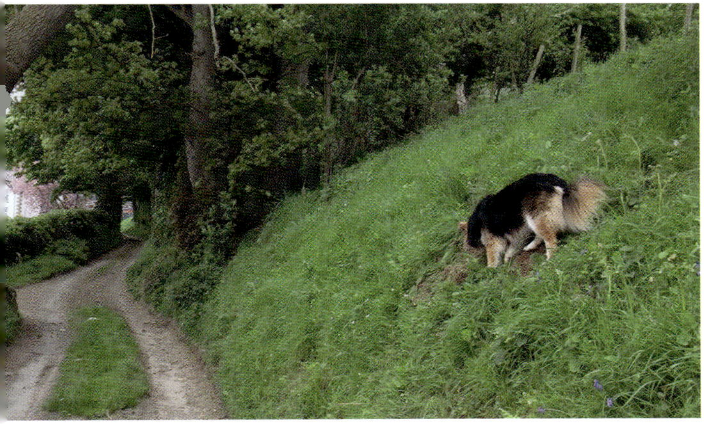

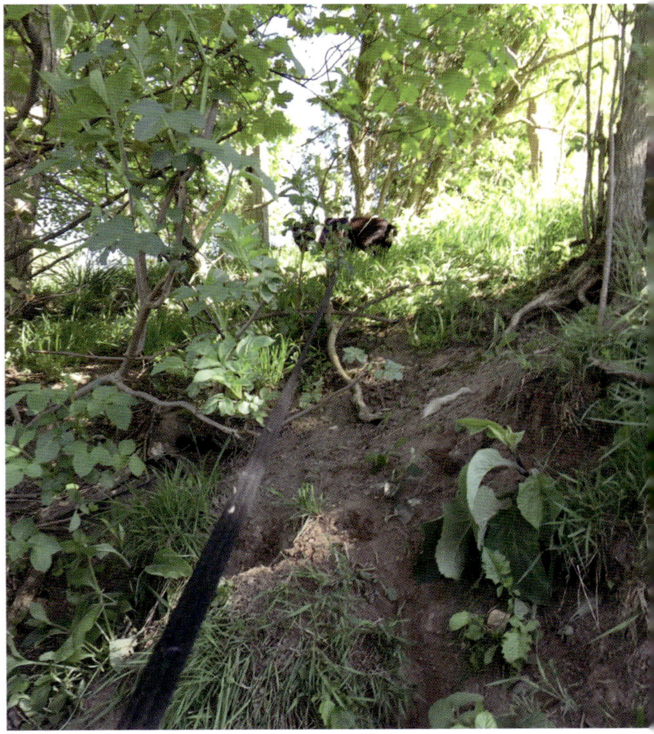

The bank was interesting for these dogs. All three were different in what they chose to do there. Notice how relaxed Pogo's body is as she explores.

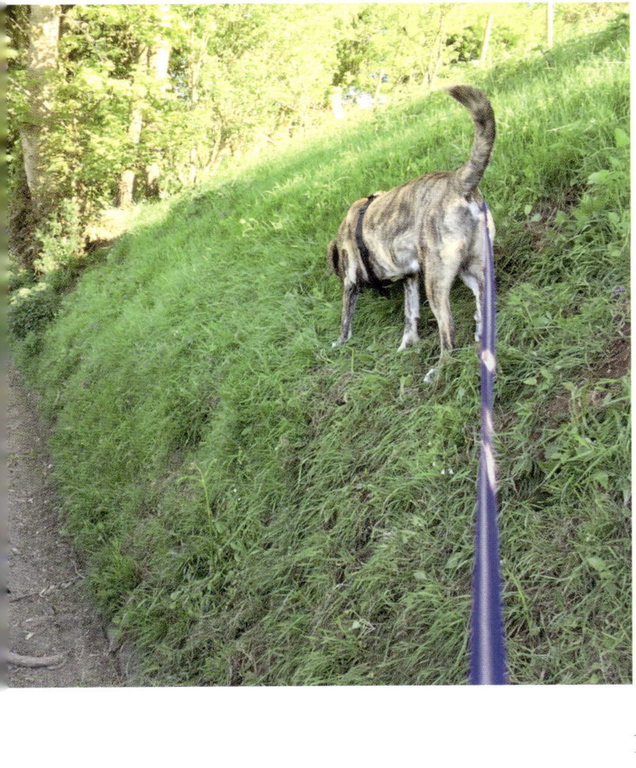

recently disturbed the hole, so there was a lot to sniff. Pogo did this methodically and took her time.

This is what I call innate dexterity. She took her time to decide what to do and chose by herself to climb the bank and take a look. I stood nearby, far enough away so I didn't invade her space, observing as we both engaged in the activity. She was calm and thoughtful, investigating thoroughly while I stood patiently watching. When she was ready to come down of her own accord, then we gradually walked back.

Nonchalantly waiting for a dog sets an example to them, as it does with people. It's also part of having a mutually respectful relationship, and over time they will want to wait for us too, meaning we have a walk together, rather than just me walking and her having to keep up.

It took a long time for Pogo to be placid enough not to chase anything that moved. Her previous life had resulted in her being in a highly-alert state and unable to focus on anything properly. These days she'll still follow a rabbit if it's close, occasionally taking a gamble on one further away, and then coming back after it's disappeared. Back then she was 'wired' and constantly on a high. However, now she's a dog who considers options, and for most this takes time to happen, especially if they're used to chasing things such as balls. Throwing balls and other objects creates a dog who is much more likely to chase squirrels, rabbits and wildlife in general. Chasing, especially if it happens regularly, can take a dog to a whole new level of excitement, from which most find hard to come down.

Another essential element of innate dexterity is about giving a dog permission to explore. Exploration encourages brain neurons to develop, although often our insecurities prevent investigation and being inquisitive. While keeping dogs safe, we also need to trust them and allow some freedom so they can find things out for themselves.

I've mentioned long lines a few times in this book and that's because they're an essential tool for us to nurture our dogs until they can be successful on their own.

To begin with, being on a long line enables innate dexterity to develop as dog and carer learn together. They need to feel and know the limits that are available, and to be able to make sensible decisions.

> By careful use of the lead, my dogs receive messages through it, so nothing has to be said; they understand from subtle information that is passed along the line, in association with my body language.

That's how they'll gain confidence, like us, taking time until we get the hang of something, and making mistakes before we know how to do it properly.

In my experience, quite a few dogs can struggle in various ways being off-lead for a variety of reasons, one being the environment may be too demanding for their skills. For some, their walks consist of being mainly off-lead. It's then that they're under pressure to make decisions and often lack the skills to do so competently, therefore getting into trouble, danger or other difficulties.

In our world, they need our help at times. Being on a long line while learning how to deal with what they encounter and at a distance takes those pressures away. Dogs appreciate this help and guidance. I can see this when Pogo asks to go on-lead, by being closer to me so I can put the lead on her and that connection helps her feel more secure. If dogs understand that help is available, they'll start to feel safe, and ask for it when they need to. I use my observational skills in anticipating times when Pogo may need intervention. This is great because it means we're working in unison.

It's inevitable that dogs, like us, will make mistakes. By defusing the situation, acting in a low-key way and avoiding reacting, it's possible to be generally supportive. Sometimes in a few situations it might be an advantage to wait for a second or two before doing anything, leaving enough time to connect with a thinking brain rather than with a reactive mind. It'll depend on the setting. Being mindful and in a good place emotionally is an advantage, because this all impacts on the dogs we're with. All of this helps to be better connected to my dogs, on their terms.

What I do for my dogs

- Understand canine communication and stress in dogs.
- Observe them mindfully.
- Give them the time they need and be patient.
- Be 'present' with them, and not distracted.
- Understand when to step in and guide at an appropriate time.
- Learn to accept their differences and difficulties.

Learning to change

I often wish I could have been able to bring the experience of innate dexterity to my previous dogs. At the time I didn't know what was happening inside them when I threw toys to chase. Using treats and training had taken them out of themselves and they weren't always aware of their surroundings, instead focused on treats and what to do to get them. I hadn't realised that all of this was fuelling them to be over-excited, which then spilled into other areas of their lives.

Over time, I learnt to see what I was doing and made changes that gave my dogs a better quality of life. When Hagrid came into our lives I was well-informed from the outset, so our relationship started on a good footing.

For my first mastiff, Kaos, I occasionally threw a toy for her in the garden. To be honest, although I didn't do this often I found it hard to stop even after learning how this activity can create stress for them, so I limited it to a couple of throws before ending it altogether. At the time, I thought she'd be bored, and felt guilty for not throwing the toy, not doing enough. That wasn't the case: in fact, she was much more balanced without the tugging toy, which not only jolted her body, but also made her extremely excited.

Kaos went on to have cruciate ligament damage in both legs while she was young. I wonder how much just the occasional throw added to the problem. I can genuinely see the damage it has done to my dogs and many others– causing psychological and physical damage.

I realise that suggesting we don't throw balls for our dogs or allow them to mainly run free off-lead could be a massive mind shift for some. After all, we've been conditioned to see a dog enjoying themselves with a huge grin and their tongue hanging out. Now I know these are signs of stress.

By not throwing toys it feels like they're not having what they need in terms of exercise, but as I understood more about stress and distress in dogs, I was able to see things differently and made changes for them. That doesn't mean they can never run or go off lead, there is a balance.

Understanding more and doing some groundwork first means it's possible to see clearly when the dog's in a balanced place.

How it is for children

Excitement happens for children and can take over. The same applies to dogs. Fortunately, the children here were accompanied by adults who intervened. However with dogs, this excitement is very often seen as play, so no one intervenes. Interestingly, the situation with the children happened on the way back from a walk, so they were tired, making them more irritable, which is usually the same for dogs.

It was a long walk, with stops and breaks and it lasted a couple of hours. Children can be tired out at home and at school, and this may seem like a benefit, giving parents much-needed time off because they feel worn out. In the long run though, the effect is opposite because it can lead to children, and adults being too tired to manage their emotions effectively.

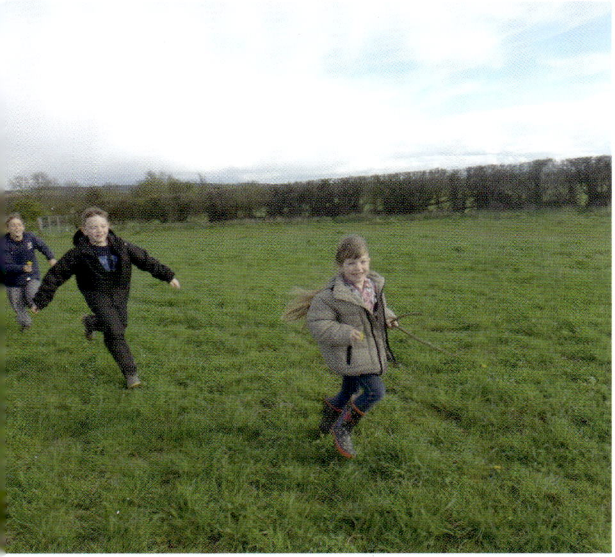

Human behaviour can be applied to dog behaviour. Here children run while out on a walk. Soon after, it ended in tears as they competed with each other, became silly and argumentative. One had a stick, which became a cause for conflict.

Here, the children are using their imagination and skills to navigate the safest way across the trees.

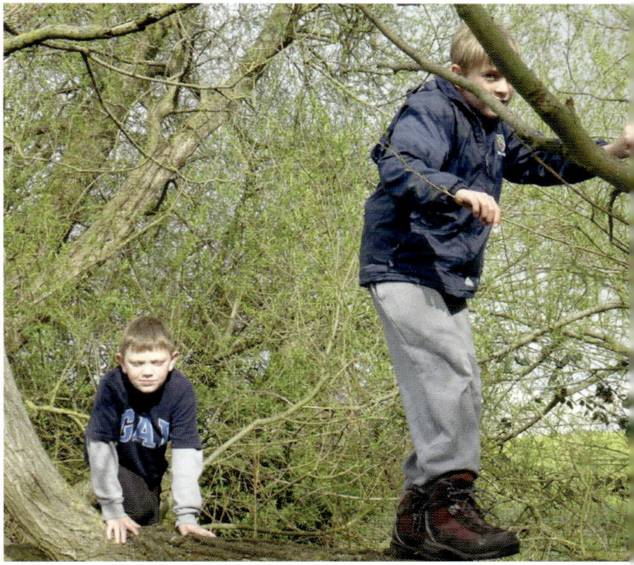

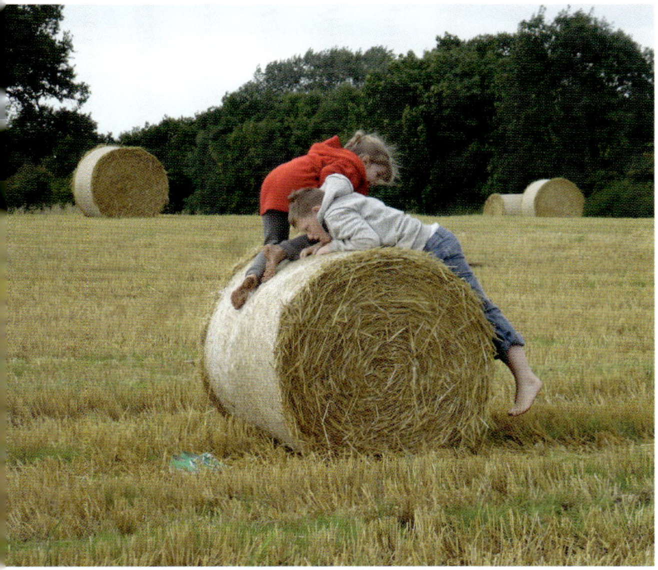

Children and dogs like to explore. The children here chose to explore, and there were boundaries. We all knew the farmer and just a simple explanation about how he earns a living was enough for them to understand why they needed to treat the bales with respect. They had the knowledge and made a choice to climb on them carefully. Like most children, if they'd been stopped altogether, they may have been more determined to do it without parental guidance and without respect for the farmer.

The children worked together thoughtfully to work out the best way to cross the tree safely. The approaches they used were different for each of them. One crawled along the branch while the other walked. Amongst other things, both gained confidence from their experiences, not to mention motor skills. They were using innate dexterity.

Adults were nearby to support and guide them if needed, so the children had a sense of being safe. This all builds connections in the children's brains. Again, there are parallels for dogs.

The same happens to dogs when they're calm and relaxed. They find things of interest, think, explore, and use their brains and bodies to solve what they face on their walk. How fascinating is that; to be involved with children and dogs as they discover the world and decide what to do with what they encounter. You're in it together.

The difference with innate dexterity to a human-centred approach is that, within reason, the dog makes choices that are supported by the handler, rather than vice versa. The dog isn't coerced or encouraged to do anything, or to explore in the way we may want him to. When a dog decides to explore, it's because they want to, and will get more out of it if it's their own decision. I leave my expectations at home when I go out on a walk. It's a subtle but crucial difference to human-led activities.

Innate dexterity in my dogs

Over the next few pages are some photos of Pogo using her innate dexterity.

There are many elements in a dog's life that can prevent them from reaching their natural inner pace; their lifestyle, the people they live with, the health of the dog, exercise and food. They can reach a settled state for innate dexterity when various stressors from these elements, among others, have been considered and appropriate changes made.

Hagrid was able to enjoy innate dexterity. For example, he could climb into a car he thought was worth exploring, or go up a bank on the riverside. He was able to seek something out in his own time and had the confidence to explore without feeling like he was going to be in trouble, locate a dead animal (wildlife), investigate the hedgerow by putting his head and body into it (just occasionally) or reach up onto manure piles in the fields.

Likewise, he'd investigate the bird table, compost heap in the garden, recycling rubbish, bins, or anything else that took his interest, within limits, and was safe for him, as in the story of him locating a cupcake and wrapper down an alleyway. Sometimes, he'd stretch himself into the car without needing to put his whole body in. On other days he'd decide he'd like to climb in. By doing so, he was able to gauge for himself on any given day what his capabilities were.

When humans lead things, we can be unaware of how a dog may feel, as seldom will he let you know if he is struggling, especially if treats are on offer.

A word of caution, however; for some dogs, the smell of other animals or food can encourage them to push themselves too much (especially if they're novel smells), and they may go to any length to get to the scent (a bitch in season for instance). As always, it depends on the dog, the time it goes on for and the intensity. Our part in this is to observe and guide as and when needed so the dog is able to develop and learn.

Dog and animal smells were always interesting to Hagrid. If his mind and body were feeling up to it, he would reach up to things to try and learn more. I loved watching him learn about life.

When a dog decides how to use their body, rather than being told, they're less likely to injure themselves. In my experience, when thinking, dogs can and do avoid things like glass on the ground, barbed wire, brambles and so forth, and keep themselves safe. They can be careful, and that's when we know an activity or a movement is suitable for that dog and that they're coming from a place of balance and grounded-ness.

Far too many domesticated dogs have arthritis prematurely. My belief is that it's quite possible to delay this and some other chronic diseases by lifestyle choices, such as the type and extent of their exercise and application of suitable limits in daily life.

Despite not being able to see well, Hagrid was clear in his communication and intent to cross the bridge. Although he found it tiring, by making the crossing he gained the confidence to be able to do it again in the future. As the years passed, on some days he would go to the bridge, choose to turn around and change his walk. He knew his capabilities, what he wanted, needed, plus I was there to guide and support his decisions.

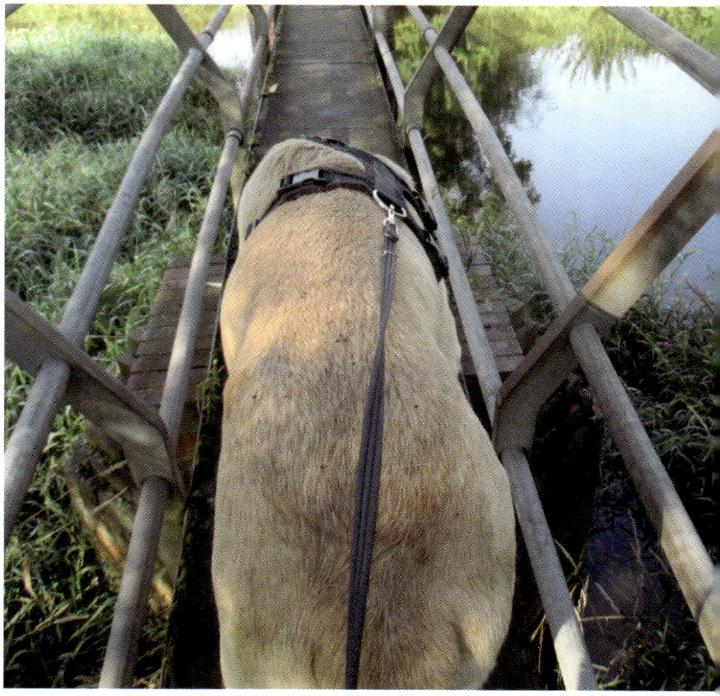

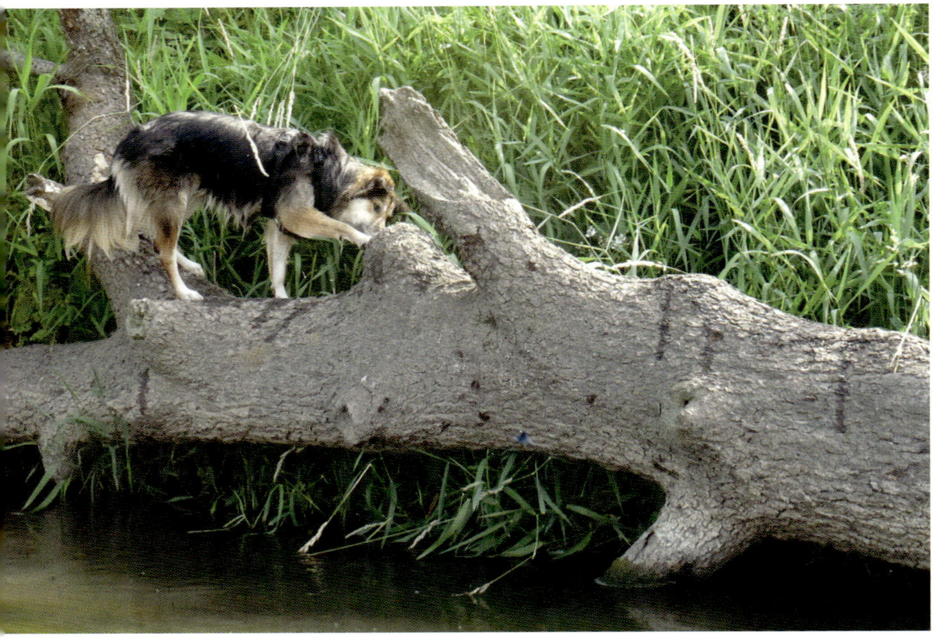

We'd been walking along on a familiar walk (one we did a couple of times a week) and so I gently unclipped her lead. Pogo enjoyed slow exploration in the river and along the banks. The way she was deeply interested in this part of the tree was a sign to me that something had probably happened there fairly recently.

One of the times Pogo was learning while off-lead. Observing her signs and body language told me that she was ready to learn without the lead for a short time, until I could see that she needed support again. Using innate dexterity, she navigated her way across the ditch. There were several ways of going through to the other field and this one required more concentration and less physical energy, but was safer than other options she'd tried before.

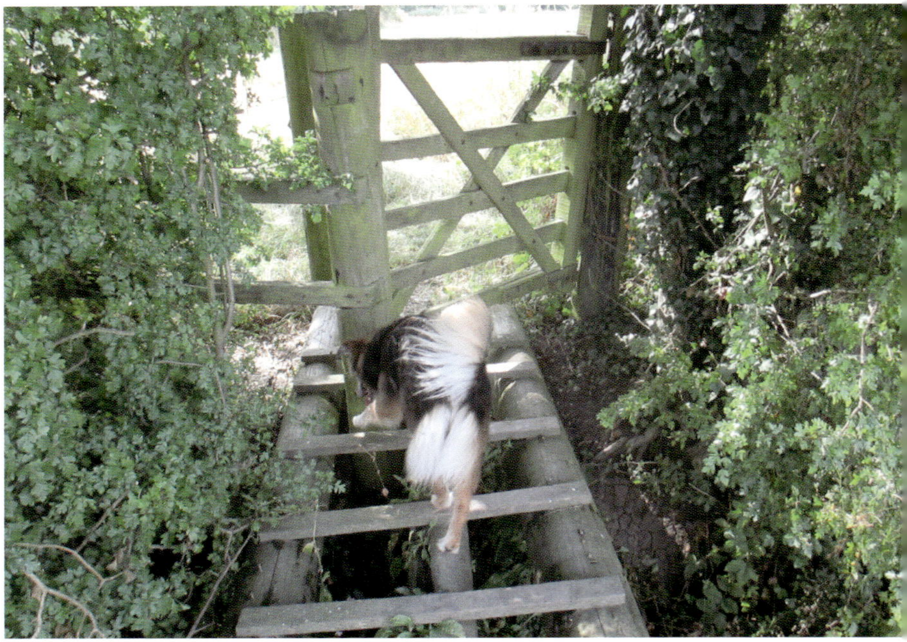

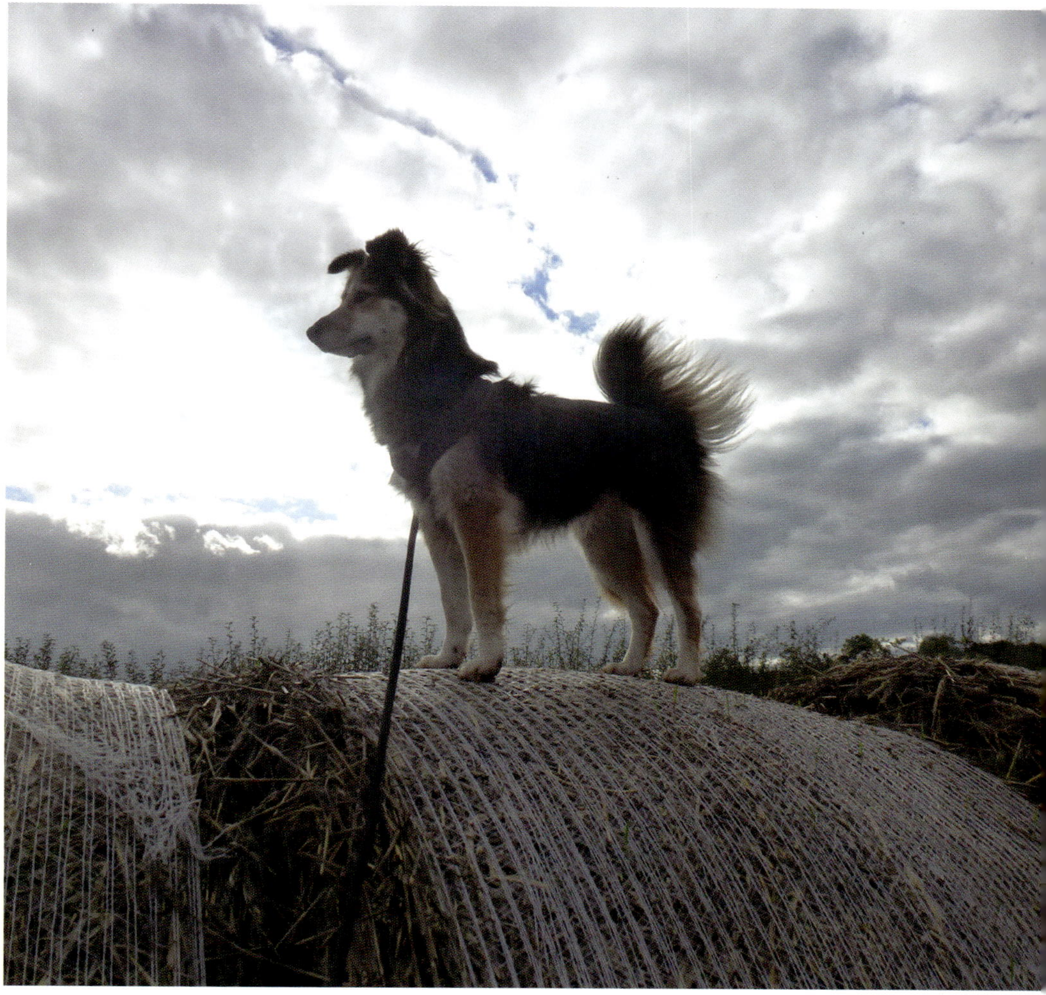

When she was younger, Pogo had a couple of negative experiences in the field next to this one. We avoided going there for a long time after, as she indicated that she didn't want to go. A few months later she seemed to be relaxed in either field. We started to come from different directions to the one where she had a bad experience, and at a different time of day, as variations can be helpful.

Someone was walking down the field. Having smelled them, Pogo jumped onto the bale to see into the next field to ensure everything was safe. It was such a sensible decision and it showed me that the incident left deep feelings over ten months later. Now, with more life experience, she rarely feels the need to check things out in this way, but she lets me know if she doesn't want to go to certain places and I respect her choices.

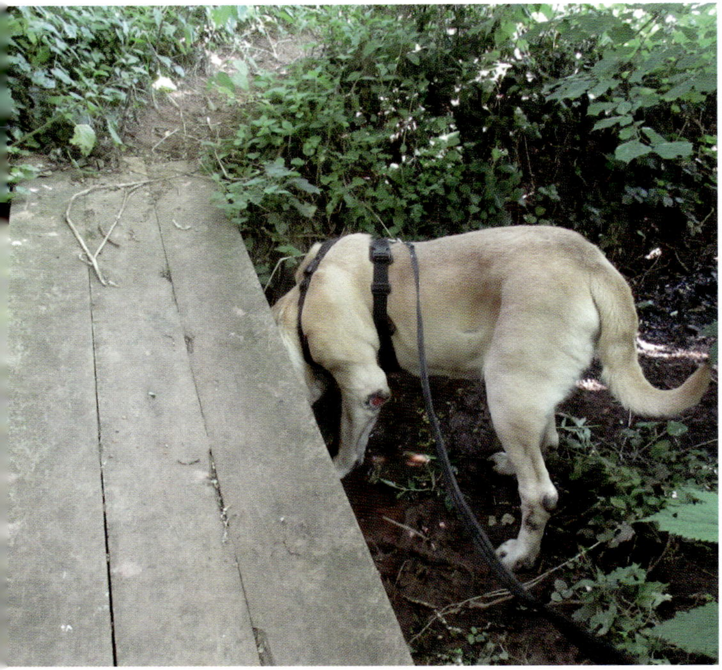

This was later on in Hagrid's life, and you'll be able to see an open wound on his front leg. Even though he was somewhat compromised by health problems, he was able to enjoy innate dexterity and continue to experience a good quality of life.

It's worth noting that while other factors come into the development of these illnesses, there's a lot that we can do to prevent or stall the chances of them developing in our dogs. Stress, environment they're exposed to, diet, lifestyle and exercise are a few areas humans can have influence over. Opting for a dog-centred approach, where the dog decides how he is to move his body through innate dexterity, will bring about a better balance than human-led activities.

Over time I've made relevant changes to our dogs' diets, lifestyles and medicinal choices based on guidance from them and it has helped them develop physically and mentally.

Some dogs might use innate dexterity on many walks, others only now and then or in the garden or house. A dog needs to be in the right frame of mind to experience innate dexterity otherwise it's something else entirely. For example, if a dog is excited in any way, their judgement becomes impaired and risk of injury increases. I'd like to share a recent example of a walk where my dog was in a good frame of mind and regulated himself well:

It was summer, raining and humid. Kuzu and I were out having a lovely walk, exploring the woods together with him on-lead. I sensed his enjoyment, he was in full innate dexterity mode as he went down a bank and examined a large badgers' set. He led me to climb over fallen trees, walk around holes, and then later, toward the end of the walk, Kuzu chose to investigate some smells coming from a field.

To get there, he needed to walk up an incline of just half a metre. A large stick was blocking his way at the top of the slope, sitting just a few inches from the ground. He had the choice to climb over or go underneath it, bearing in mind that Kuzu is a big dog. To my surprise, he chose to squash himself on the ground and wriggle underneath. This was a message to me that he could be tired, too tired or uncomfortable in some way.

After this, we chose to go back to the van. Kuzu was tired and was able to make the best choice for his body. This is what happens when dogs come from a place of calm and they can make appropriate decisions based on their ability.

When a dog is off-lead and regularly rushing around for any amount of time, adrenalin kicks in and they can make unwise decisions which they may end up paying for later, especially in the long term. Some may start limping straight away, others after they've rested or had a good sleep.

Taking the above as an example, let's imagine for a moment that Kuzu was off-lead. He'd have been much more likely to jump over and clear the stick, and I wouldn't have realised he was tired or uncomfortable and over exerting his body. We may have kept on going with the walk, further exhausting him and potentially creating issues.

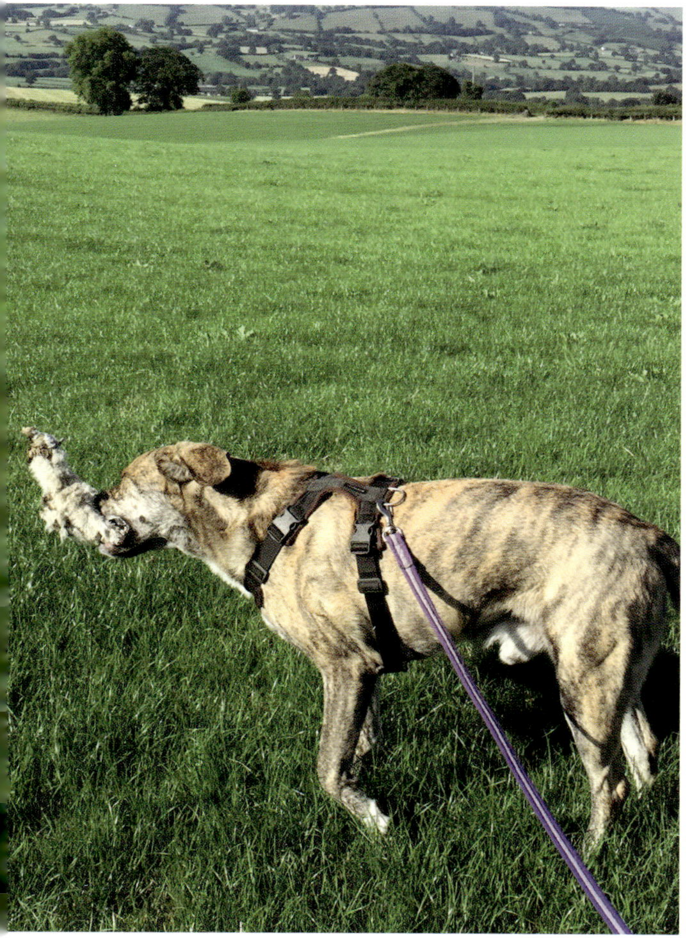

Here, Kuzu found a dead animal. He decided to chew on it and eat a little, then after a few minutes he left the rest of it, moving on to explore something else. Allowing animals such things comes with risks, and it wouldn't have been possible for Kuzu to have these kinds of choices when he first came to live with us. He was underweight, undernourished and food-obsessed.

Now, because he's satisfied with his food and balanced in this situation, he can have a little and leave some. Indeed, sometimes he doesn't need to bother with them at all.

A word of warning: dogs can be at risk with anything they do, it's up to us to know our dogs and put in boundaries ahead of time when we think something isn't appropriate for them.

The sad thing is, without awareness, dogs can be worn out. People do it to themselves, at the gym or at work, and could then have problems sleeping or resting. I have experience of pushing myself too hard and each time it's resulted in anxiety, being 'wired', and always seeking more. On the other side of this, their innate dexterity has the potential to keep dogs mentally and physically active for years because they're working within their natural limits, not overworking themselves. This then leaves them in a good position to be able to have quality sleep and rest.

Shadow, is making choices on a relaxed walk. He took his time to find the best place and way to turn around to get back along the tree. A delicate procedure. It's possible to see a dog grow in confidence, which impacts on other parts of their life, mostly their overall mental health.

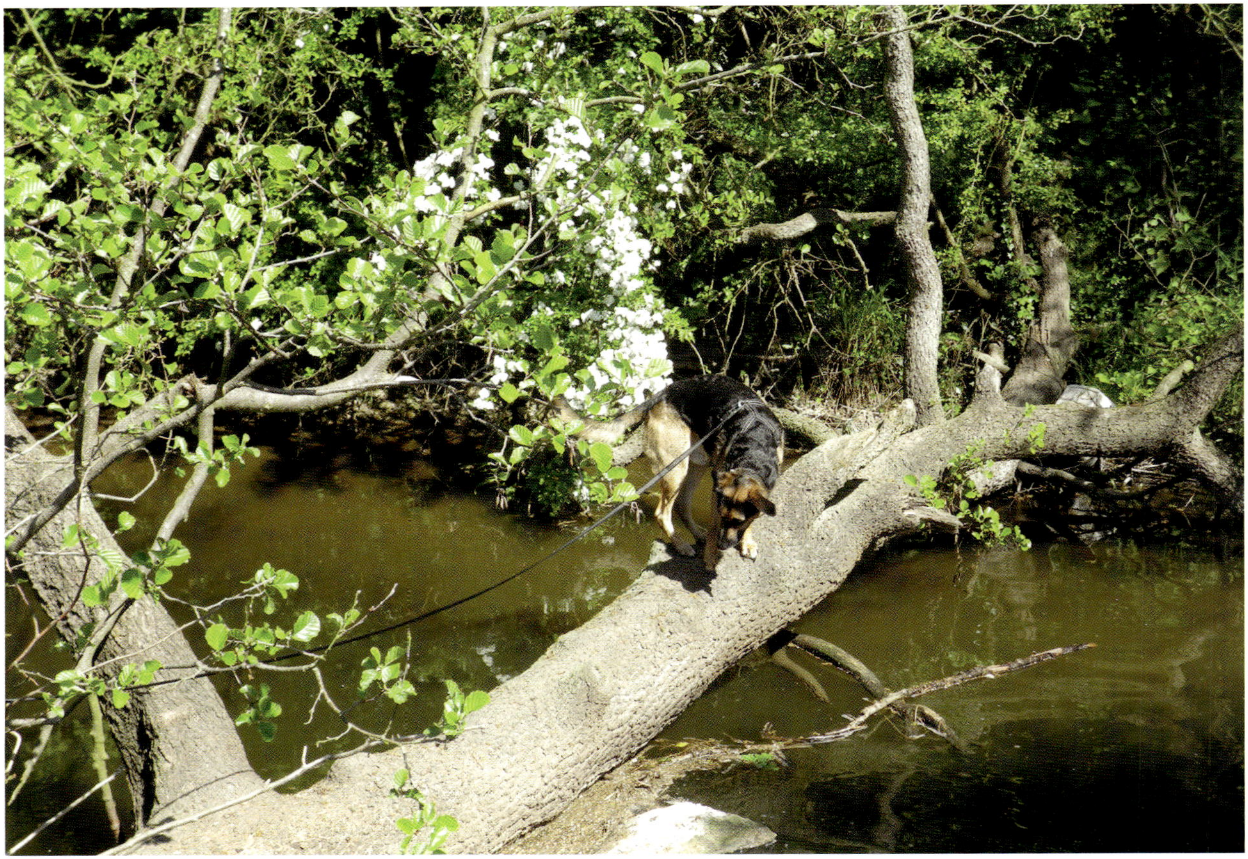

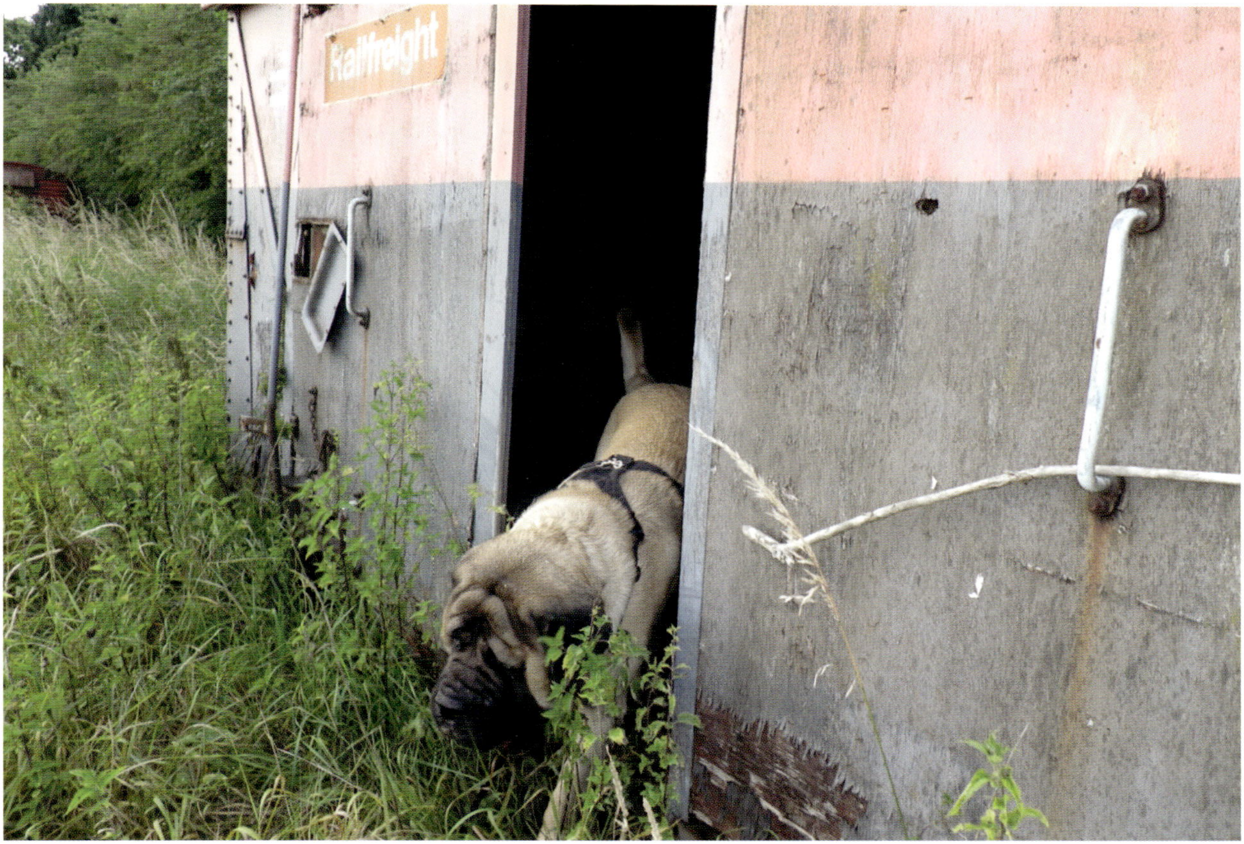

In summary, innate dexterity is when a dog has the freedom to explore, make choices and use their body how they decide to. This is from a grounded place, with a grounded handler, and together learn about each other while feeling the connection through a long line as they navigate a suitable environment. But most importantly, the dog gets to make their own choices, within set limits, that then develop into having more options in life.

The health benefits of innate dexterity

- Making their own choices, supported by their handler, allows the development of new neural pathways when able to make these choices regularly.
- It builds confidence.
- They can become calmer and more balanced over time.
- Dogs learn to recognise their own capabilities.
- It gives their body and brain what they naturally need, working in sync.
- Mind and body stay well for longer because of the avoidance of overexertion.
- It enables the dog to have quality rest after a period of activity.
- On the whole, there's less stress and pressure from us on the dog.
- It builds the bond and trust between dog and carer/handler.

Chapter 18

Intrinsic reward

When a dog comes into a new home their immediate need is to feel safe, secure and loved while they grow in confidence and relax into their new surroundings.

For this to happen, they generally require plenty of time to just 'be' and become familiar with what's going on around them. After this point, they're ready to learn and slowly expand their surroundings, gathering new experiences and then returning to the environment they feel safe in.

I know I felt proud to have a dog who did what I asked and dogs who are obedient will do a trick on command and can certainly give us a boost in our own confidence. This is how I used to feel when I trained dogs. It was quite a powerful feeling to know I had control over them, which I mistook for them liking me and us having a good relationship. I was paying them, in a way, to do what I wanted without much consideration or really getting to know them in the true sense. What I've learnt over time though is that these tricks do little for the dog in terms of helping them to learn or develop the life skills for staying safe and handling social situations.

I'll elaborate on what I mean shortly, but first I'd like to take a diversion on a little trip to the gadget museum! (See *Further reading* for details).

Bear with me for a moment as there's an important lesson in here, I promise.

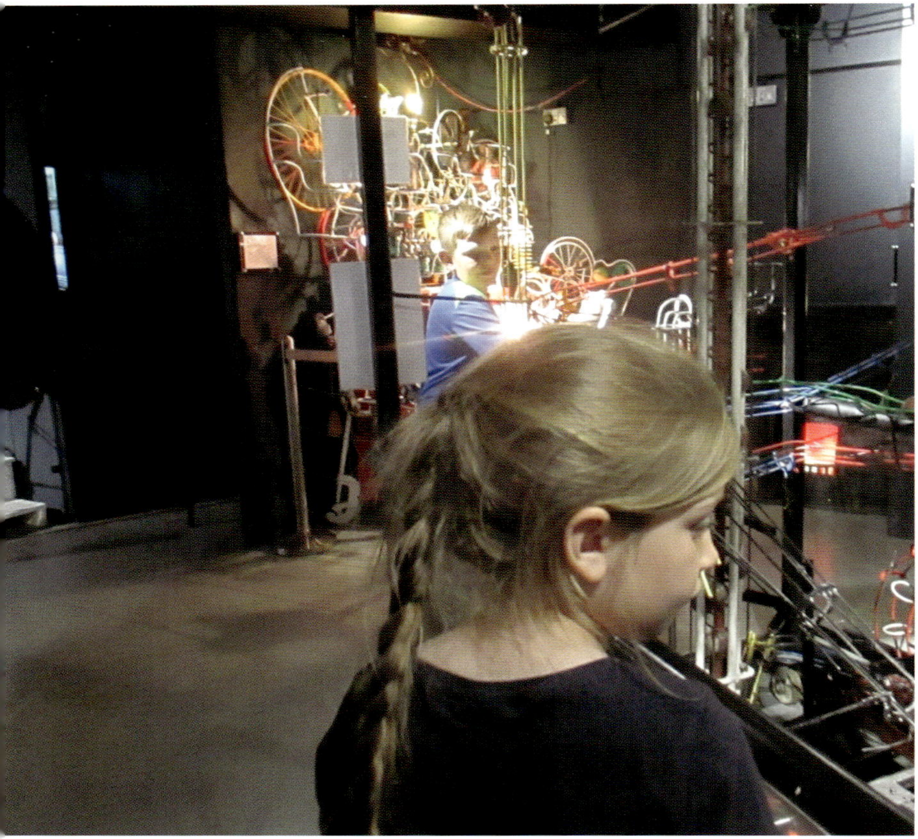

At this point, William and Katey were enthralled and curious about the machines, what they did and how they worked.

to win. It was such a shame to see this change.

We tried to explain to them that by slowing down to operate the machines, they'd still be able to find the figures, rather than rushing around and missing them. Instead, the children were overexcited and hadn't taken the information in because they were only focused on the reward at the end.

Eventually, having searched both floors of the museum twice, and finding all but one figure, the children were rewarded.

As soon as we arrived, the children became engaged in a shared interest. From my point of view, it was truly lovely to see them *genuinely* interested and asking questions. But this changed once they were told about a prize at stake for identifying twelve figures that were hidden on the gadgets. Competition between them overrode everything else, a frantic urgency to find the figures developed, the interest in the gadgets went and they became selfish, wanting

The interest and curiosity that was there in the beginning which took time, required concentration, developed important life skills and encouraged them to want to learn more about the gadgets wasn't there now; it had been replaced by the drive for a prize. What the children had learned was how to be quick and not focus on the important things or their natural curiosity. They were paid to do a quick job and were bought.

Research by Dr Kristin Neff and her team[1] has shown that people can achieve far better results by developing self-compassion and self-determination when doing things that offer an intrinsic reward (something rewarding in itself), rather than merely working to satisfy an external drive. People who work to receive accolades, rewards, bonuses and recognition usually discover that the satisfaction gained is short lived and they quickly find themselves chasing the next prize. Whereas people pursuing goals based on mastering something for themselves rather than performance are measurably leading a more purposeful, satisfying and fulfilling life.

How does this relate to dogs?

When translating this to dogs, we can see that when being trained with treats, toys or other motivators, they act in a similar way to how the children did in the museum. The dog tries to work out "how can I get the reward?" and "what's in it for me?" rather than being able to enjoy whatever they're doing.

Dogs, like many of us, feel good about themselves and gain confidence when given a choice, as long as it's within their range of skills, otherwise it can be too much for them. The best reward for a dog is one they've taken time over; it's mentally stimulating and satisfying, and provides them with skills for real-life scenarios. I've learned this, and now that my dogs aren't given rewards I realise how in the past their focus was on the treats. Although they needed to work out how to get the food, they weren't learning anything useful. It was centred around what *I* wanted and making life easier for me. In a genuine relationship that works for both, where you consider one another, you don't need rewards to make the other one do things.

Instead, dogs learn that by complying with what we want them to do, they get something nice, which interestingly often interferes with them needing to communicate to another dog or people. By complying, they become more dependent on us – which might make us feel good – but is this fair for them?

It's possible to have a relationship where a dog is able to have choices to do what *they* want, within safe boundaries. I love seeing this and observing my dogs deciding what to do in different scenarios. They're free to explore, within reasonable limits, the way they do intrinsically, without needing to stay around just in case there may be a treat on offer. When we're out and they're off-lead, they tend to walk within a certain range while exploring, occasionally going

1. Kristin D. Neff, Ya-Ping Hsieh and Kullaya Dejitterat (2005) Self-compassion, Achievement Goals, and Coping with Academic Failure, Self and Identity, 4:3, 263-287, DOI: 10.1080/13576500444000317. https://self-compassion.org/wp-content/uploads/publications/SClearninggoals.pdf

further for a few moments and returning when they've finished. It's all quite relaxed.

Of course, people usually like to have their dog fairly close to them and have the ability to recall them, sometimes using treats, so it can be scary at first when the treats aren't there to fall back on. To begin with I could even get panicky if I didn't have dog treats on me.

Using rewards is much quicker and easier than working on building a two-way relationship and trying to understand a dog.

We can pay people to want to be with us but how real is that? I changed things with my dogs because I wanted to understand and know more about them, their character and choices, on all days and that's my intrinsic reward; getting to know them for who they are, on their good days and bad days. I'd like a friend who chooses when to be around, to be themselves, not a dog I have to pay to be with me.

Teaching a dog to sit is quite complex. Sitting is part of their language and for some it can be a sign of comfort, while at other times it's an essential part of their interactions with other dogs. Some are uncomfortable with this position, especially for any length of time. Dogs can also struggle with other positions we ask of them. When left to their own devices, they may sit for short times because they want to, or to send a message to another. It can put them in an uncomfortable or vulnerable position if they've been asked to sit, especially when around other dogs. In these situations, a sit suppresses their emotions and interferes with what they need to convey to other animals.

By asking them to do this in the presence of others or in delicate situations (to them) we could be interrupting their conversation and responses; one that we may not understand or be aware of at the time. When this happens it's asking them to do something that may be completely inappropriate at that point in their conversation. From their perspective, however, they just don't understand why it's important to sit right then.

Think about the reasons behind why a dog is asked to sit. I've not asked any of my dogs to do this for many years, we've got by just fine and never needed it. They sit as and when they chose to. Is it so important to ask them to do this, or is it something we've just become accustomed to seeing and asking?

For a significant number of dogs, rewards put them into another mindset; their attention is falsely elsewhere. They can seem urgent and frantic at times: "give me the treat", solely focusing on that. With some of the dogs I used to train, it was so obvious. However when they went into that mindset of "what do I need to do to get a treat?" I felt sorry for them, as they were so anxious to do the right thing that produced the treat, often making mistakes, being clumsy and oblivious to what was going on around them as they tried.

The scientific link below is related to this topic:

sciencedaily.com/
releases/2019/05/190514093420.htm

Often children, adults too, are treated in a similar way, encouraging them to learn and behave through rewards. This can produce adults who lack the confidence to make decisions for themselves, and so make poor choices. Adults who have difficulty making their own decisions without a given goal, tend to suffer from depression and anxiety problems. But sadly, few people are able to recognise the signs of this in dogs.

Rewards and punishments create conditional behaviour, and while treats are much nicer, they're still used for gaining control through coercion.

When dogs are used to making their own choices and problem solving, they get an intrinsic reward from that. They learn and understand much better having worked something out for themselves than if they were just manipulated using a reward such as treats. Without the use of rewards and given the right amount of distance, Hagrid was able to look at other dogs, and make sensible decisions. In time he learnt the appropriate social skills to be able to assess a situation.

Previously, when he encountered a dog, he'd perform a play bow (but what many people don't realise is that in this case it meant he wanted to exit the situation), then become over animated, unable to use his thinking brain. This was because he hadn't yet learnt to problem-solve, despite the fact that he'd been surrounded by many dogs for the first few years of his life. He'd learnt some coping strategies that enabled him to survive in the overwhelming living conditions he had no choice but to endure.

Do you feel an intrinsic reward when you have worked something out for yourself rather being told to do something? I certainly do, it's the best thing, although there are times when I look for guidance, usually while still learning.

While they're learning skills, offering guidance and support to dogs is essential for their well-being. Although it is true that many will know better than we do in some situations they understand, they will require help because, up until this point, we're likely to have made the choices for them.

It's possible to help them, as I did with Hagrid, by not putting him into situations which he didn't have the skills for at that time.

And of course, what better intrinsic reward is there for us than observing and learning from our dogs? They tell us so much when we're ready and willing to step into their world, and only then we can grow together.

CHAPTER 19

Enhancing a dog's life

What we did with Hagrid to enhance his days during wellness and illness

Throughout Hagrid's life we did quite a few things with him to add enrichment, in spite of his uneven health. Often quite simple things mean a lot to a dog; energetic activities would have exhausted him and added to his problems. There's a balance to be found, and sometimes it may not be recognised. Less is more, and that goes for the majority of dogs, more so for young, elderly and sick ones.

Hagrid enjoyed exploring friends' cars, especially those that smelt of dogs, and also visits to various houses where he mooched in rooms downstairs and explored the garden. Friends and family would bring enrichment. One friend, Jean, would kindly bring back items she'd found on the beach for our dogs to investigate. Something we do is to have bags of interesting items for our dogs to go through. My friends and I regularly swap bags of appropriate items and the dogs are able to pick up each other's scents and information about one another.

Sometimes Hagrid would take the bag, open it and go through by himself or I would disperse the contents and then let him have a look. I have found using enrichment to be really useful and it can help some dogs. Most dogs get a lot out of this time.

Short treasure hunts were fun, although long ones can be too tiring. I'd lay a few items around along the route the dogs would take, making it easy enough for them to be successful. Occasionally one or two objects would be placed slightly higher for the dog to find, in and around stones or mixed with sticks and leaves.

A few items used:

- A box of balled up paper with something inside.
- Recycling rubbish that's safe for the dog.
- Upturned plant pots with a small piece of food underneath.
- Bedding from another animal.
- Old discarded clothes.

When doing this, it was interesting to observe when the dogs came across the items and what each one chose to do; and if they didn't want to interact with them, that was fine. I didn't point them out, it was for the dogs to explore at their own pace or not if that was their choice. We can learn from them. After they had finished, everything would be cleared up.

If one of them had found something difficult, I'd make it different the next time. Usually when Hagrid found something he recognised, he'd wag his tail in recognition, then walk on. Nothing major, but that was his way of reacting.

As I've mentioned, I rarely use treats with my dogs. Sometimes it's fascinating to see how they take notice of what they find without involving food. Please see the chapter *Intrinsic Reward*.

Occasionally, I do a similar low-level activity inside the house with a couple of boxes containing a small

Hagrid would enjoy exploring a friend's car who regularly had different dogs.

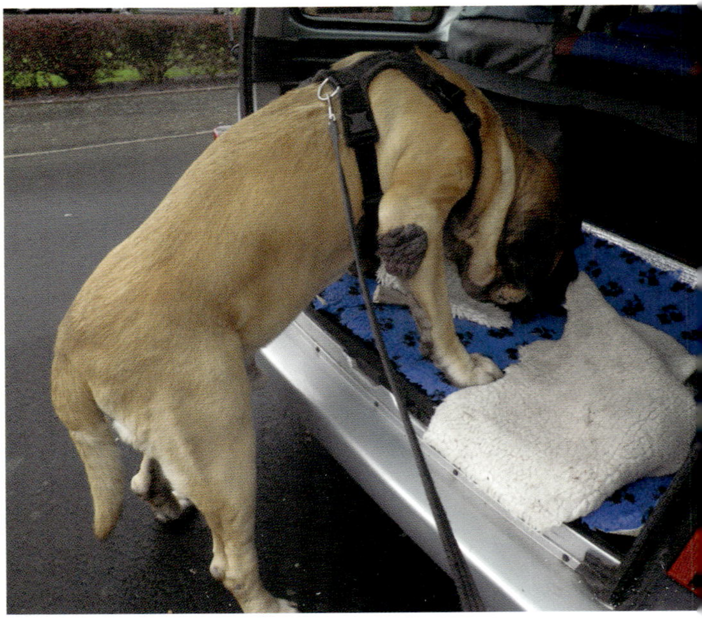

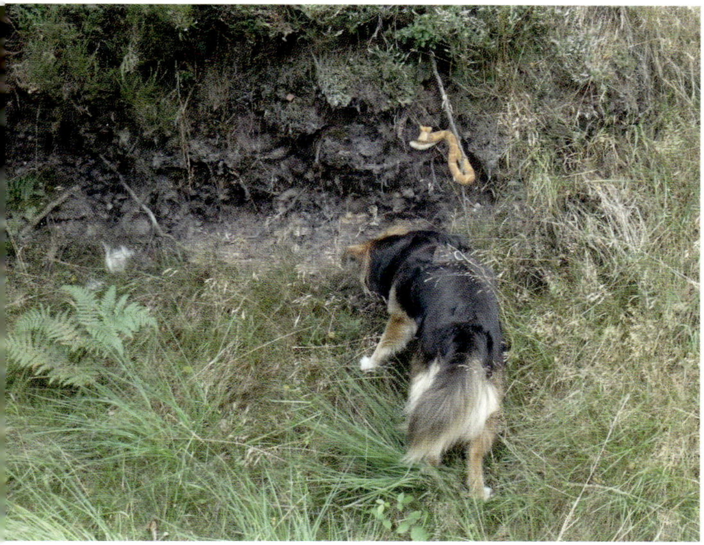

Pogo sniffing out treasure near the orange toy snake. For this part of the treasure hunt she was able to be off-lead; her experience and skill level allowed for this. For other parts of the walk, she benefitted from being on-lead.

healthy treat wrapped in paper, placed around the house for a dog to find in a quiet and gentle way. My dogs take their time to look for things without the need for a cue, meaning they are able to think about what they are doing and work things out for themselves. There's no pressure on them to find anything, so if they don't seem to realise, it's just left there. Sooner or later they'll sniff it out in their own time.

I am careful to avoid situations where there could be competition because there may be a problem if one finds something and the other doesn't. That can happen when food is involved, if not managed adequately. Thinking it through first is what helps, so each dog has a chance to find something, often in a different part of the house or garden.

Enrichment

I bring items back for my dogs whenever I go somewhere; dog beds from friends' houses, seaweed and other items found on the beach, bits and pieces from farms, including bedding from other animals, fur, feathers, wool and so on, whatever is around. Once I came across a bin bag of clothes that Hagrid found fascinating. After that first time exploring them he continued to find the clothes really interesting for a few days afterwards each time they were brought out again. All of this added so much interest to Hagrid's life.

Safe items from charity shops are always interesting for dogs and these can be passed onto friends with dogs, cats and other animals for their enjoyment and scent to be left on them. Our cats and rabbits spent a lot of good time investigating the dogs' enrichment, which was interesting for all of them.

As mentioned, Good friends Marilyn Aspinall, Jean Gough and I regularly swapped items of interest for all our dogs, and once a month or so we'd meet up and have a walk somewhere with some or all of them. All the dogs had regular updates about their friends via the bags of enrichment we swapped.

Getting used to a dog's smell is the first step to them becoming familiar with each other, and this is how we went about introducing them.

We ensured a careful introduction over time, so that all dogs became familiar with the others, within their comfort zone. Taking it slowly helped to create a harmonious relationship. The dogs can take their time to get to know one other, first by smell, then at a distance, and if appropriate, close up. What often happens is that the meeting turns out to be a non-event as both are already well aware of each other; they often amble along together sniffing, occasionally sharing the same smells.

I've noticed it's worth keeping a careful eye on how the dog reacts to the different smells as some can cause distress, and not all dogs are suitable to meet. Not all dogs will like another's smell. Sometimes it's possible to see them take a wide birth around a patch of ground or some other scent, indicating a definite dislike.

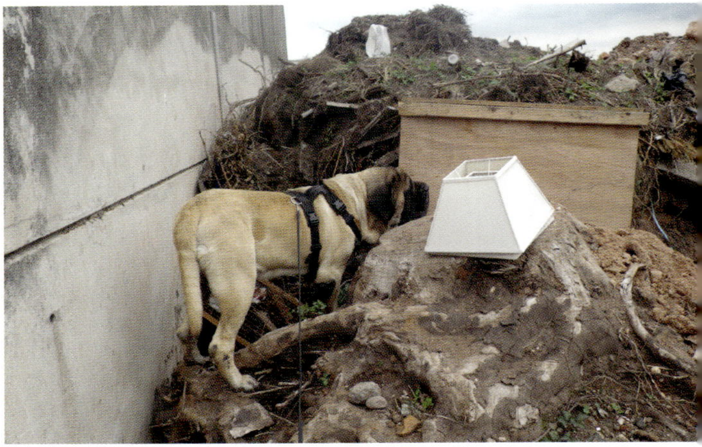

Although not far from our house, we drove to this place and walked a few metres where there was a dumping ground that Hagrid found extremely enriching. He was able to climb up to different levels if he chose to. Once there was an old rabbit hutch there, as shown in this photo and so many other items that offered interest for any dog.

Branches we brought back from a walk with another dog, which gave Hagrid some interest.

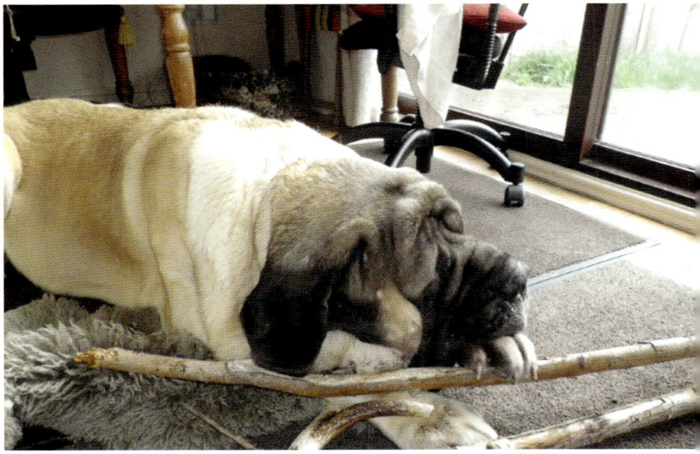

A visit to the river, on-lead. Time spent just being there and paddling or sitting down ensures that Hagrid didn't over-exert himself.

Water was something he loved and it did over-excite him early on, but in time he adapted and was able to enjoy time near the river, especially during the summer months.

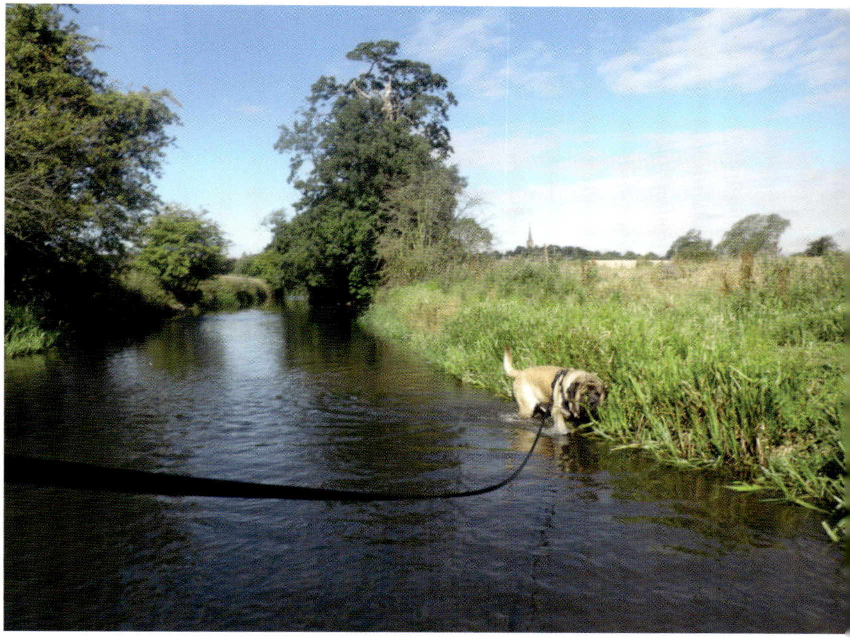

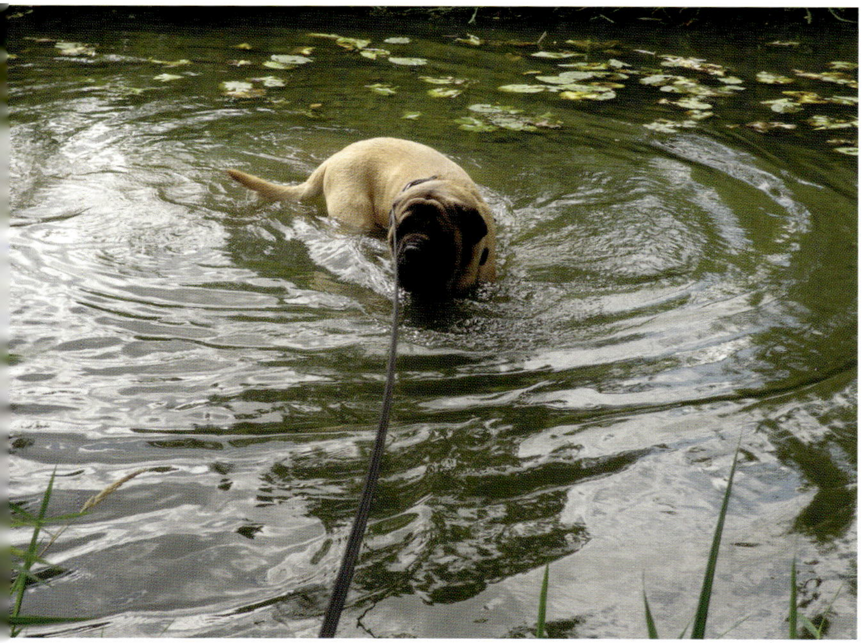

Coming back after the boundary had been applied was something Hagrid understood clearly, from use of the lead. He came back after a few seconds. Used in this way, a long line is a wonderful teaching tool.

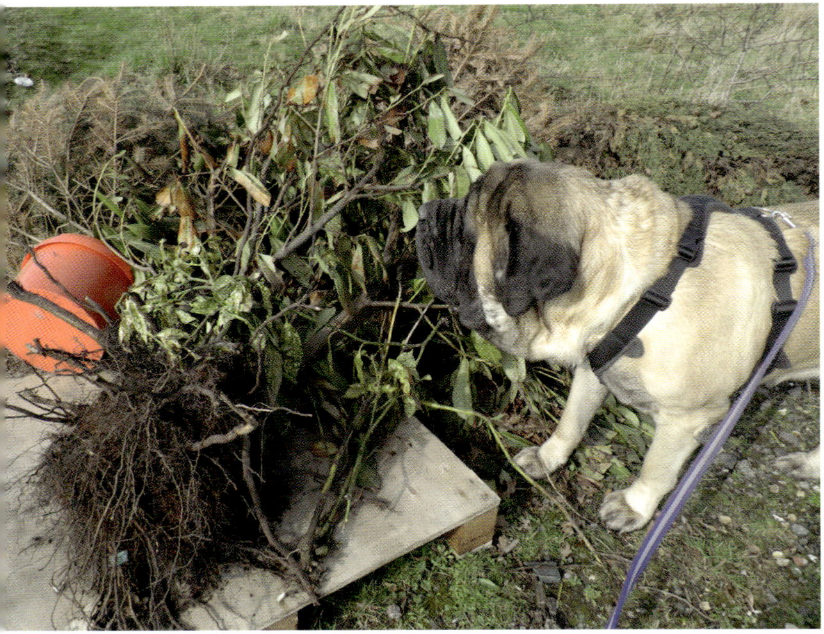

Items discarded at the back of a garden centre.

A take away coffee cup found in the garden centre car park seemed to be the bargain of the day and Hagrid took it home with him.

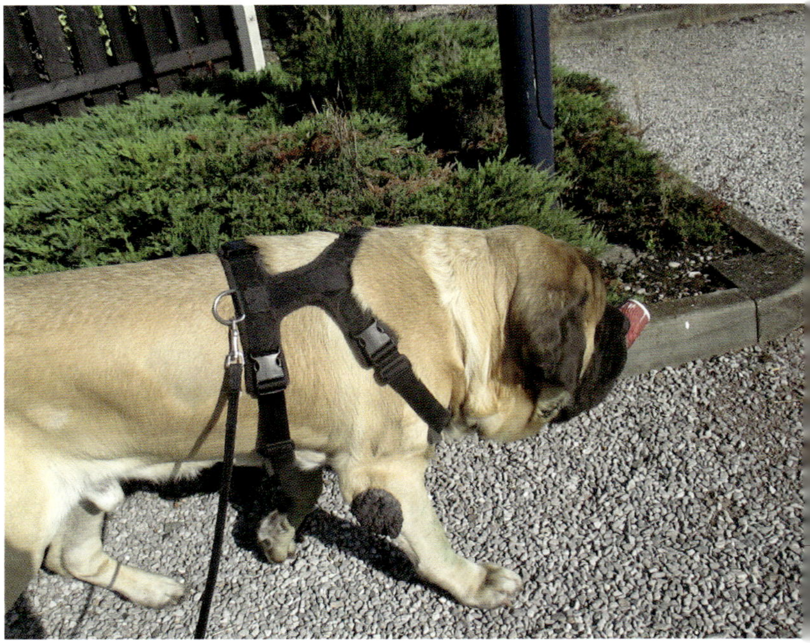

Occasionally we visited the local Garden Centre that had a big car park, where one end was hardly used.

Hagrid found much of interest, especially discarded Christmas trees, furniture where people had sat to enjoy drinks; just so much variety here for a dog.

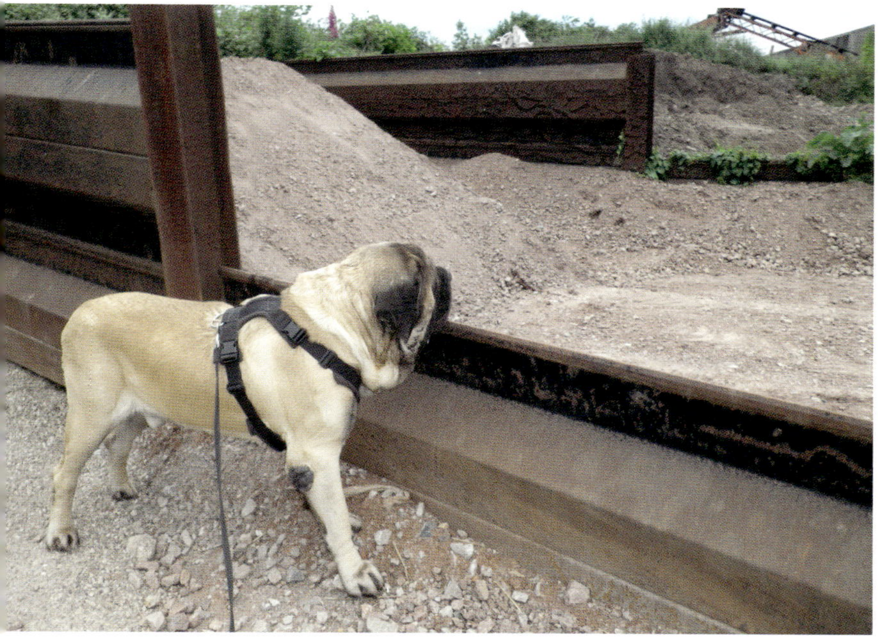

Can you imagine the interesting smells here?

Quite varied experiences in this farmyard. It was possible for Hagrid to see things from a distance before approaching. Then over time he could get closer as he gained more confidence and familiarity. Again, going slowly was the key.

One place I regularly took Hagrid toward the last few months of his life was a farmyard that was also used as an industrial unit. He had many good times there.

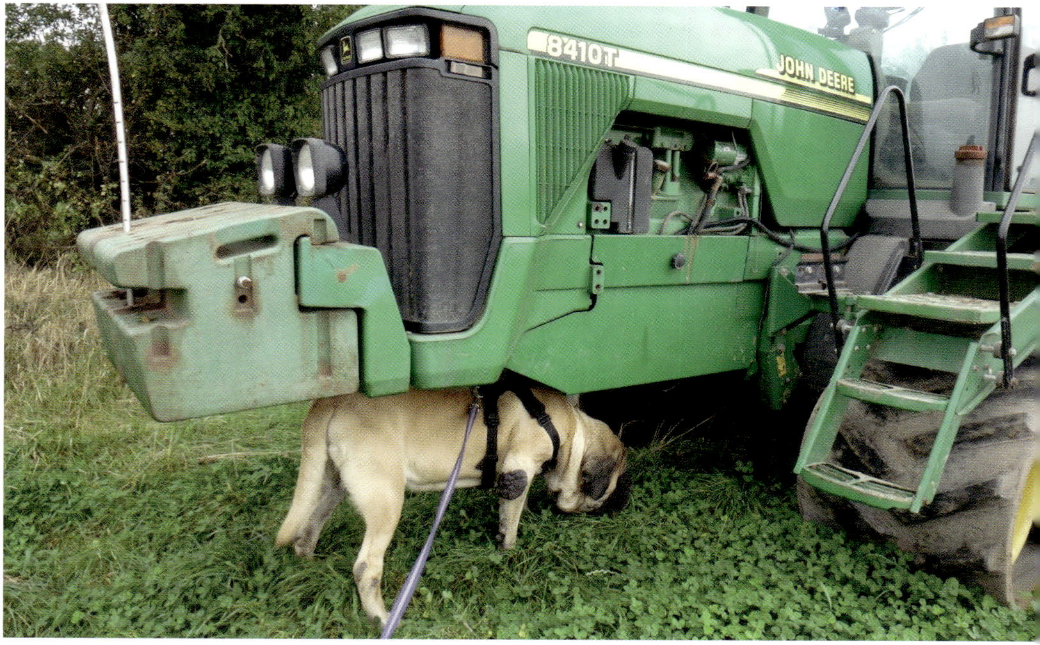

Stacks of tyres were homes for mice and rabbits living in the area. There were farm buildings to explore; places where the hay and straw bales were stacked. I asked permission to walk Hagrid there prior to going, and found people can be really helpful once it had been explained why the area was of benefit to a dog. Being on-lead was a requirement: people are more likely to trust that their land will be respected.

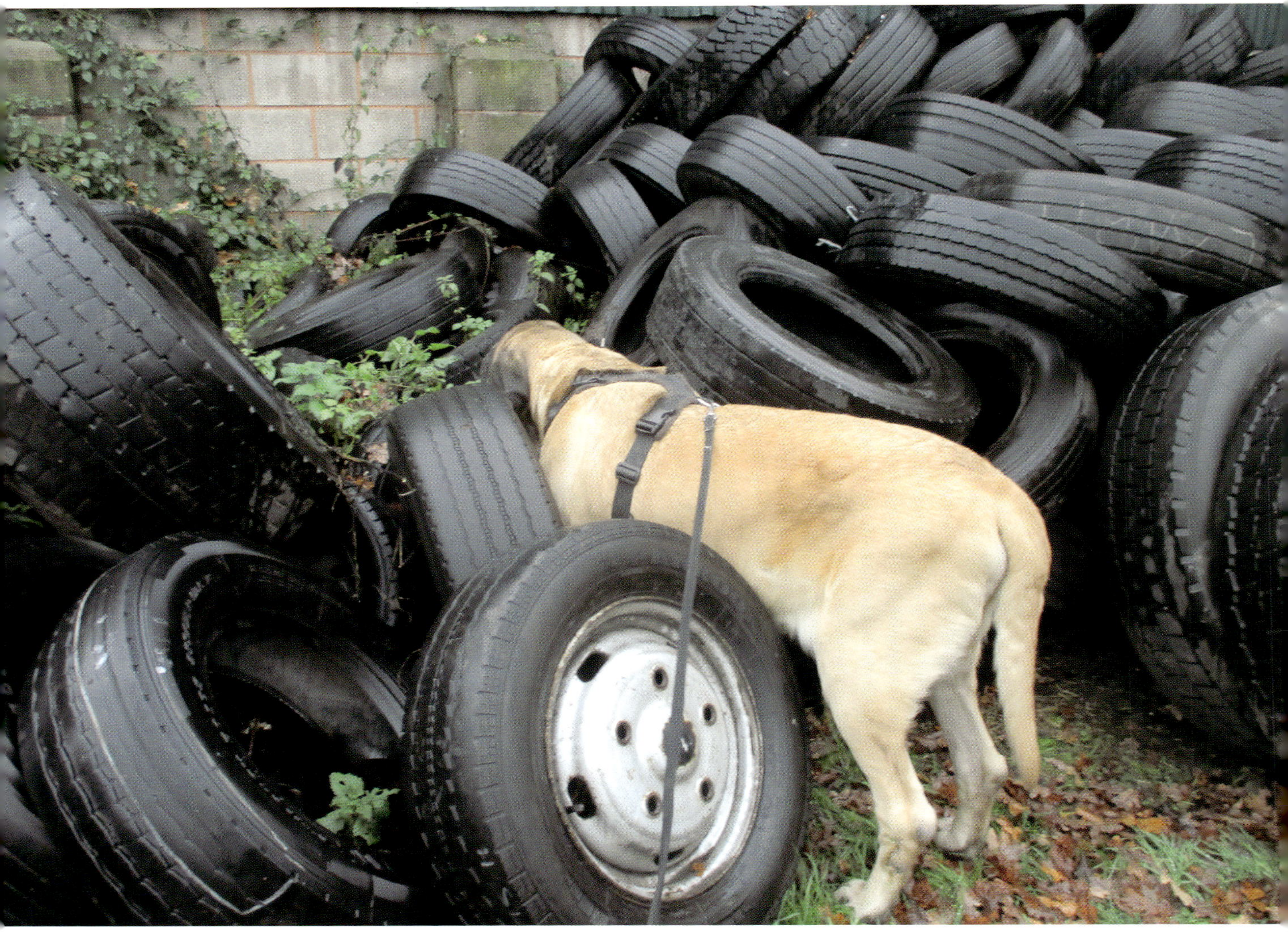

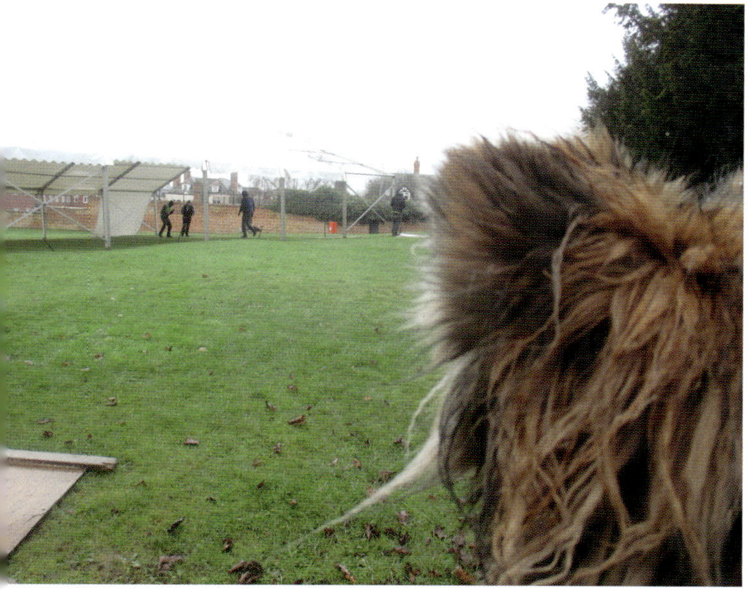

On a familiar walk with Pogo, a French market was being dismantled so we took the opportunity to sit and watch for a while. We were used to sitting here and watching, and this day there was more going on. Pogo loves just watching like this.

In the past it helped her to understand the world without being involved, which is when her emotions would have been heightened. There was lots of interest here and being far away from what was going on was ideal. It had been a busy market for the couple of days before, meaning that there were many smells in the area for Pogo to sniff. Most dogs are quite content staying in the background and having a natural interest without all the attention that people usually like to give.

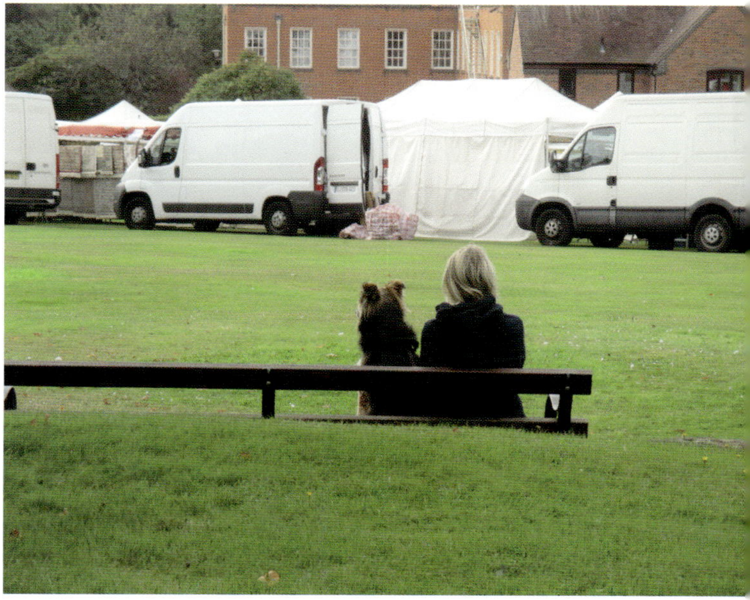

Then there were times when we cleared the garage out and our dogs explored the piles of things for keeping and throwing away. They were involved with the whole process and told us when they'd had enough by going back inside to lie down. These kinds of opportunities gave them the chance to use their brains and have some physical exercise; climbing onto things, looking inside, going under chairs, lying down to chew on something they'd found, and so on.

Hagrid would come around while we were in the garden doing jobs, and after a short time he'd lie down and sunbathe on the patio. He loved to be out in the garden and, like most dogs, enjoyed just being around his carers. For a sick, old, or for that matter any dog, this can be valuable quality time.

Having building work done can be challenging for dogs with the noise, disruption and strangers in the house. I made sure that the dogs felt secure in these unusual circumstances by keeping them and the workmen apart. I asked and the dogs always had a chance to explore the builders' tools while they were having lunch and after they'd gone. At these quiet times it was a chance for the dogs to make sense of what was going on.

These simple things gave them information about who was in the house and then they don't necessarily need to meet them.

There's so much interest for dogs in life, and it's simple things like this that can make their day, when they have time to look and sniff at what they find.

In time, after asking them, one or two workmen would just carry on with their job and Hagrid was able to sniff while they were there. More great, positive experiences of people being happy to help, when approached in an open and respectful way. All these times added up to outweigh the negative view of people, which he had before being with us.

Visits to the industrial estate gave Hagrid opportunities for exploration in a safe environment. As I've said before, it's important to know what a dog is likely to do with what they find in these areas before going. Hagrid found it really fascinating and was able to have a quality walk there.

These areas can be fairly quiet at times and some of the rubbish is involving for dogs, as it was for him. Amongst other things we found discarded mattresses that were safe and a skip where Hagrid could sniff the rubbish that was on the top. We could be there quite a while, and this was another opportunity for him to encounter people at a distance while they were working.

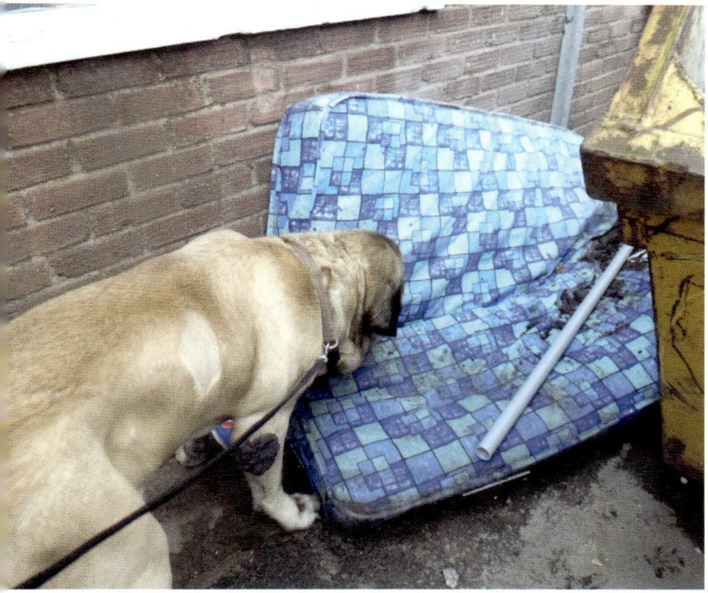

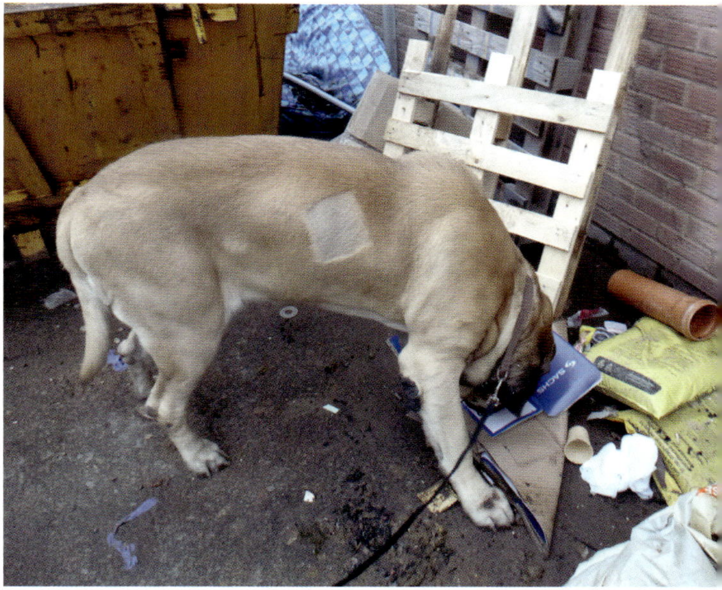

There are opportunities everywhere that hold interest for a dog in the most unexpected places.
It's easy to pick up the spilled rubbish afterwards.

Before the bins were collected I'd take Hagrid round the block. This was a special walk where he inspected the neighbours' recycling rubbish.

It took a while to get around and I did put boundaries on the lead when applicable.

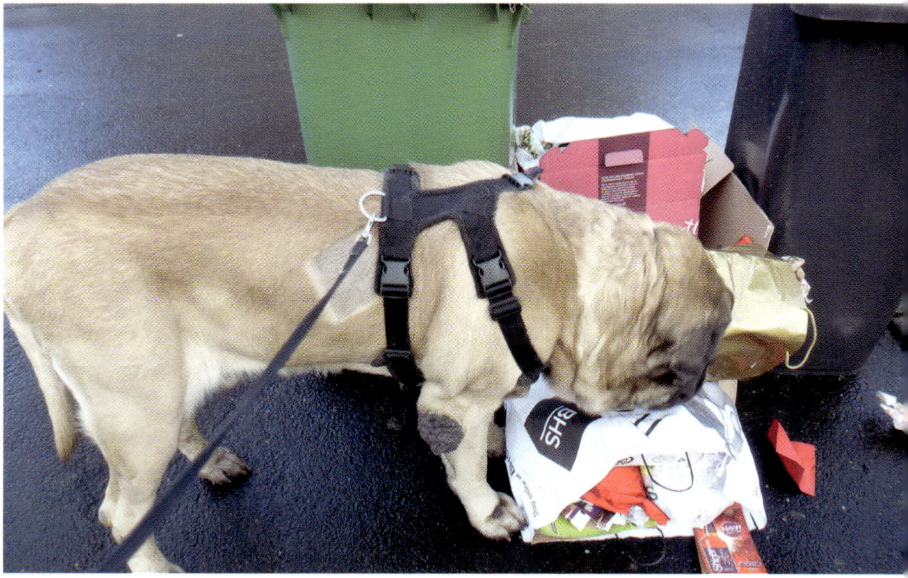

Visiting places where other animals were around is another stimulating thing to do. So Hagrid met cows, and they came walking over to see him each time we went, which was one of Hagrid's favourite walks near the end of his life. Then there were horses who also came over to sniff him, and donkeys and sheep too.

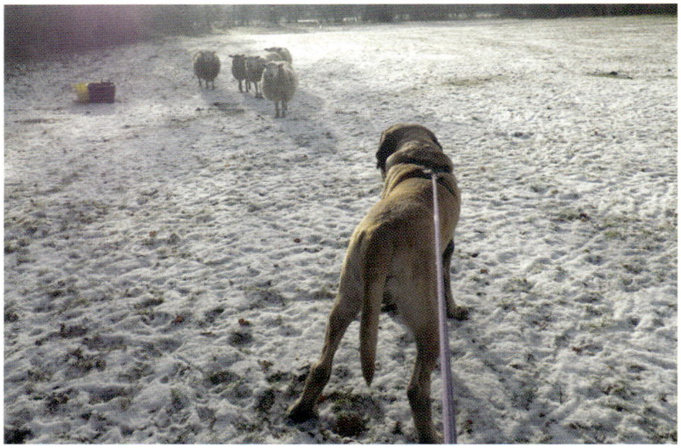

The lead is used as a boundary, giving Hagrid thinking time and a message that that's close enough. Given a few moments Hagrid turned away from the sheep - a sensible choice.

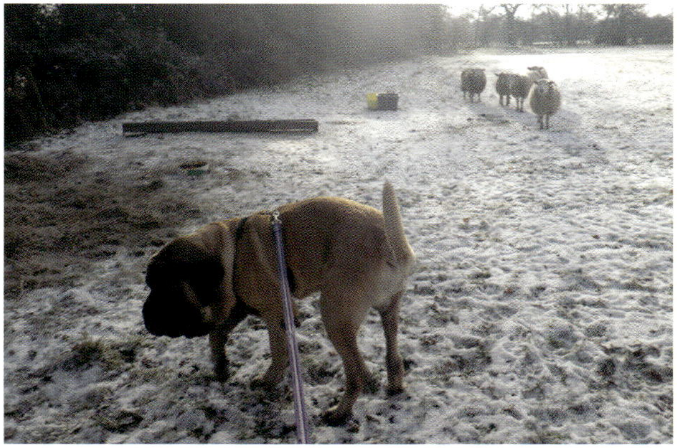

Sheep that walked toward us when we went into the field! Can you see the slight curve to his body? Hagrid was inquisitive and wanted to go closer. I decided to go back so he could see them from behind a gate, with a boundary in place. There was a clear stop applied on the lead, with no need for me to say anything to him. Hagrid decided when he was ready to turn around to come with me, which can be quite a difficult thing for a dog to do, especially in this kind of situation.

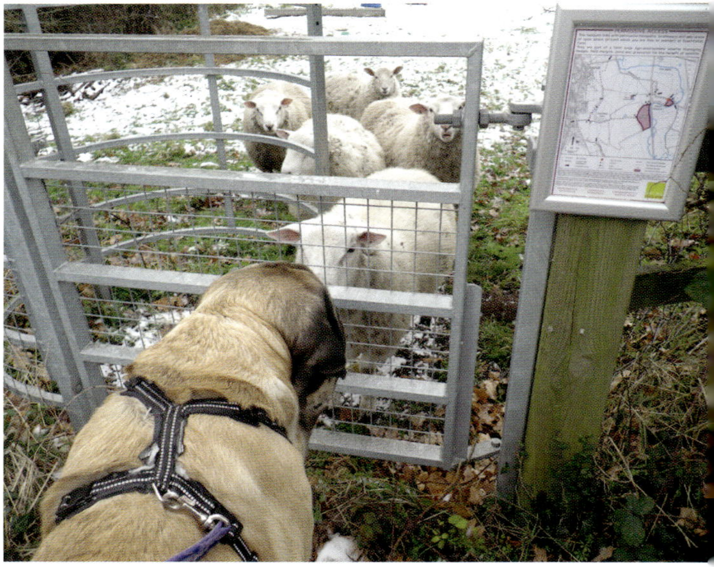

They sniffed each other behind the safety of the gate. He was quite intent on meeting them in the field, which told me it'd be safer from behind the gate. When a dog is really intense it can scare other animals and as I knew Hagrid, that was close enough. He'd met sheep before at a large distance. For a positive experience for all, it was best to have a barrier or a good distance.

Hagrid was a dog who had daily struggles, but he also had lots going for him. Although he didn't often go far, and at times didn't always go out for walks, that didn't mean his quality of life was compromised. He enjoyed sniffing around, seeing cows in the fields, spending time with the cats, paddling, lying on the patio, sitting and watching life happen, relaxing with classical music playing, and all those things made his life worth it. I know he wouldn't have wanted to die before he did, and I actually wonder if a few more days may have been what he wanted.

We managed the pain, and when the medication didn't work I looked for different ways to manage it. There were times in Hagrid's life when he was uncomfortable and in pain, and life can be like that for humans too. It's my belief that as long as there's hope, there are possibilities to get past these times. I'm not saying it was always good, but for many years there really was hope.

Looking back at all these photos, Hagrid was often somewhere filled with interest that wouldn't always be evident to the human eye. There's usually so much close by us that offers stimulation for dogs without it being too much. Just take a look at cats when they're outside and the things they do. They spend a lot of time watching, doing little things here and there, but generally living a slow, contemplative life. Dogs are similar when we're not involved and a scenario where they're more in control, like cats are, is nice to create for them.

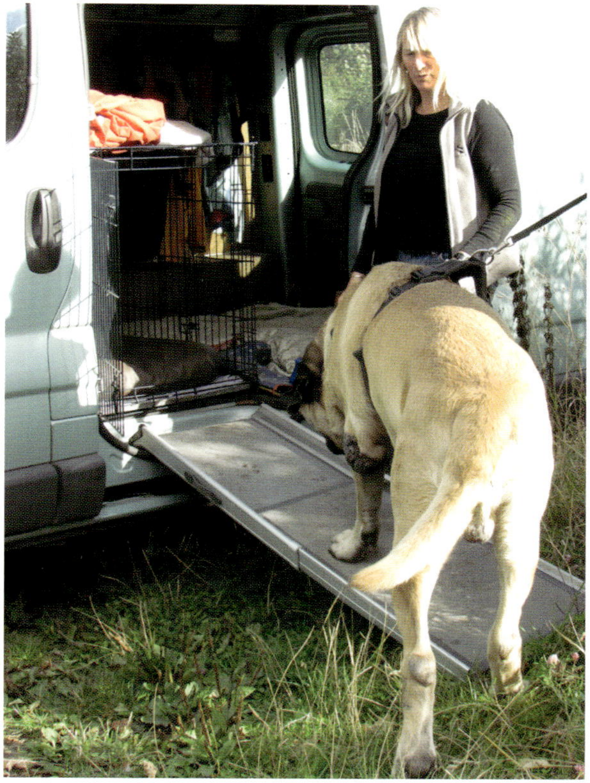

Adjustments to make life easier for a sick, ageing dog can help them to deal with life comfortably. Using a ramp and guiding Hagrid onto it was an essential part of his freedom to choose. Because he had trouble with his eyesight, we're using the lead to guide him up the ramp. If you notice here, the lead is tight and that's what he needed to feel secure.

When you start thinking about it, it's actually quite easy to make the most of the kind of opportunities I've talked about here. They're everywhere for you and your dog to discover.

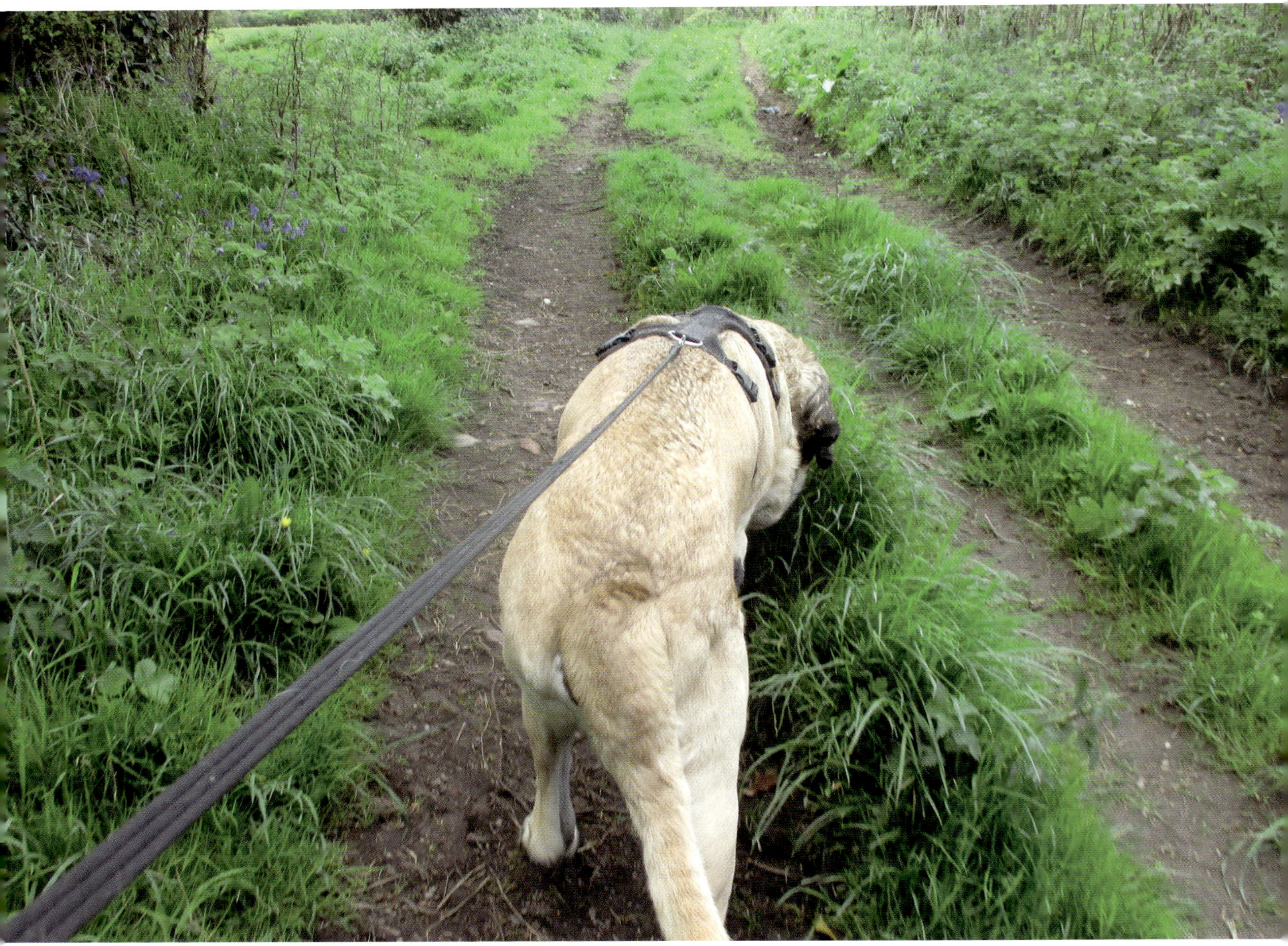

One of Hagrid's favourite routes. He was always so interested in sniffing around here. I have no idea why, what he could smell, but it was an attractive, enjoyable place for him. We had many happy times there, and in the surrounding area. It was easy to see anyone coming down the path, giving us enough time to move away into nearby fields if needed.

Key points

- Short treasure hunts were fun for each dog, although long ones could be too tiring.
- Home-based treasure hunts for healthy treats were rewarding, but thinking it through in advance, so each dog had a chance to find something in different parts of the house, was beneficial to avoid competition.
- Whenever I go somewhere I like to bring interesting items back for my dogs so they can relate to where I've been; dog beds from friends' houses (to return at a later date), seaweed and other items found on the beach, bits and pieces from farms including bedding from other animals, fur, feathers, wool and so on.
- Our cats and rabbits spent a lot of quality time exploring the dogs' enrichment, which held interest for all.
- I've noticed it's worth keeping a careful eye on how a dog reacts to various smells, as some can cause distress, and not all dogs are suitable to meet each other.
- Taking things slowly helped to create a harmonious relationship.
- Clearing out the garage gave our dogs the opportunity to explore the piles of items we intended to keep or throw away.
- Visits to a local industrial estate gave Hagrid opportunities to explore in a safe environment.

Epilogue: hope for a wider shift in awareness

Shortly after Hagrid's death, I was out having coffee and a lady across the table from me asked what I was reading. It was a book about dog behaviour. We began to talk a little about dogs and I asked her what breed she had. She said she had a spaniel. I love all dogs and previously shared my life with spaniels, so naturally I told her how lovely I thought they were.

She replied by saying that they weren't lovely, and told me that her spaniel was deaf and had ear and skin problems. She went on to tell me about the nightmare she was experiencing with her dog. The dog had been on steroids and antibiotics for five years.

"Five years!" I thought. I found that shocking. It was what she said next that I found encouraging.

Apparently she'd had enough of the medication and took matters into her own hands. Over a long period of time, she'd gradually weaned her dog off the prescribed drugs, without telling the vet. The lady also mentioned that she'd moved house, and although she didn't say where to, it was a much quieter way of life and didn't have to walk her dog past traffic anymore. Due to this, and perhaps a few other factors, the dog was better than she'd ever been, and her coat, lost as a result of taking drugs for so long, had begun to grow back.

I need to emphasise that generally it's not a good idea to take a dog off medication without consulting your vet. Working with a vet to establish a good relationship while the dog's communication is taken into account is what works best. It's also in the dog's best interests.

Maybe the lady didn't know that giving her dog a quieter life would help overcome some of the health issues, but she had insight to recognise why the dog had improved. I too, couldn't continually rely on antibiotics and steroids with Hagrid; I just felt it wasn't right for him so did my best to avoid them whenever possible, only using them when absolutely necessary, once other options had been explored without success.

Although I don't know her or her dog, this information was given to me without the woman knowing anything about me and what I do, so it was interesting how on par with my philosophy she is.

This story, the result of a chance meeting, gave me hope that in the wider world people are looking for options, using complementary as well as conventional treatments, and thinking about improvements that are based upon intuitive wisdom and knowledge.

This is the heart of what my project in this book and in my wider life has become. I want to make the dynamic clear: there is veterinary, behavioural, and cultural knowledge, and then there is our own intuitive understanding from our emotions and experiences. Because of the way this knowledge has developed over time, in many situations it's much easier to take the word of science and practitioners over our own understanding and to the exclusion of that understanding. In so many scenarios I have felt I have to take the line 'I will do what you say because I trust that you know better than I do' so that we can, for example, have surgery, take medicine, improve our mental health, do the right thing socially, and so on. And all of these things are beneficial.

It's really why we're at where we are now as a society, but looking at people I see plenty living on low quality food in an unsuitable environment, and many are on some kind of medication, which can easily diminish their long-term quality of life. Life expectancies are longer than other parts of the world. But what does that mean and is a long life everything? It's very sad: my own mother is living a long life but she is unable to care for herself and doesn't know who she is, or anything about who she used to be. I believe she still has some degree of quality to her life although her choices have been taken away. There are lots like her and there will be even more in the future. I don't want to be like that for myself or my family.

Already I have years of making poor choices, until realising the need to take responsibility for my own actions. And you're reading about some of what I've learnt along the way. Making balanced decisions that are best for us at the time is so important to our overall well-being and outcome and, along with other factors, each decision we make is our future.

The effect of this, though, is that because of these situations where I feel we have to defer making decisions, often dismissing our intuition, a culture has been created where people are likely to ignore what they think and feel intuitively about certain things, and completely trust advice given by science.

I think in a wider sense as well, this has led to an approach to life that is reinforced socially by attitudes, where the first step is to distrust our intuitions, not take them seriously, and the second step is to automatically trust the advice given and treat it seriously.

In my experience, doing more relaxed work with dogs, trying complementary therapies, or even changing my diet, I've come across some who do not take me seriously. They doubt what I'm doing because it's based on a combination of observation, experience, study and responses to how I feel intuitively, coming from my own understanding. Indeed, how many times in this book have you felt your own reluctance to accept something I've said because it hasn't come from a scientific background, but from my own experiences as a human being? I think fundamentally people are reluctant to trust themselves when it comes to their own well-being or their dog's.

We live in a culture where we are expected to do what we're told, despite professional advice not being completely flawless, and intuition not being completely unreliable.

How many times have you heard of cases where medical professionals have given incorrect advice and misdiagnosed? Or how many times have you heard of someone's intuition and self-belief about health being correct against professional judgement? My father died after a mistake by a doctor, being told for weeks that what was ultimately cancer, was a hernia. This was followed by a further mistake in the operating theatre, which led to his haemorrhaging a week later. His usual consultant confirmed that the operating theatre mistake wouldn't have happened had he been there and not on holiday. The point I'm trying to make is that by working together, with all positions being respectfully considered, professional advice and intuition have a role to play in a holistic approach.

In my experience, however, it isn't just mistakes by professionals that contribute to the advice given being an incomplete solution to problems.

The science is good, in fact science really is our intuition built upon and investigated to find a more controllable way of using what we're picking up intuitively. I've found that often it's the application that doesn't always quite fit with what it's repairing. I've mentioned this in the chapter on vets; much of the problem will be the difficulty of the application itself.

With the limited time available, a vet can only really build a snapshot of the possible causes of the symptoms being shown by a dog, especially when a symptom on its own can be an indication of not just one but a whole variety of problems. Largely, they really do a great job. I feel the problem is one of insufficient time and information. Life can be rushed. In these situations, there is a fine line between giving suitable and unsuitable advice. Because carers have a daily experience of what is happening in their dog's life, that input can be valuable. Vets do ask, but as mentioned, the time constraints make the job more difficult.

I'm generalising here: I believe that often, for some, the combination of a lack of faith to make decisions about all kinds of things in life, along with unreasonable expectations of others who we see as more legitimate to be able to tell us what to do, boils down to how we treat those who we're responsible for; namely our children and our pets. I believe it's true to say that, in society, quite a few people feel the need to tell dogs what to do at every point of their lives and ignore what a dog might want to do, because they can't be trusted, they can't be taken seriously, they're just dogs, and we know better because we're smarter.

Maybe you've felt uncomfortable with the ideas I've talked about earlier in this book of allowing dogs to choose where they walk or what they eat, within their capabilities, because they can't be trusted with these decisions. But I have seen from my own experiences over the years, both in terms of learning to trust how I and my dogs feel about things, that this position of extremes, of completely trusting one and ignoring the other, is not the most effective way to lead our lives, either for health or happiness. The point of this book is to show there is room for a more balanced approach.

There is such an incredible depth of understanding and knowledge that is naturally within us, both people and dogs; whether that is being able to sense that something doesn't feel right, or to make decisions based on emotions as indicators of what is and isn't good for us, or to directly express what the body needs, as with self-selection.

As with choices for dogs, the first step is to restore the ability to listen to ourselves, as many of us will have ignored it for a long time; then to try and decide from this what is and isn't useful, because of course like science, our intuition isn't perfect either, and any of us can make mistakes.

I believe, however, that to apply any of these ideas about redressing the balance between outside advice and internal information to our dogs' lives, we first have to embrace it ourselves. To show a dog trust, I first had to be able to trust myself.

> It takes two to have a good relationship, and to be in balance, because whatever the carer is feeling the dog will sense.

Dogs benefit from the same freedoms that we do. Dogs want to be able to have choices as we do. They want to be able to be trusted as we are. These are natural things that go in to make up a healthy, balanced life, physically and emotionally, for carers and for animals.

The first step is to give them value, to believe that there is more to them and accept them as sentient beings. This is probably the idea that's been met with the most social resistance. Some people can be sceptical, even annoyed, by me taking dogs seriously, treating them with respect, cooking and preparing food for them, offering them choices, walking them individually and being there for them. I know not everyone will have the luxury of time, yet I believe there is often scope for adaption that can be made to further understand and benefit the dog.

I think most people would like a close, easy, unproblematic relationship with their dog that consists of going on good walks, being friendly, easy-going, and happy. And I've learned that by trusting and considering them, giving them choices, respecting their communication signals and understanding that they are dogs living in our world, it's possible to build such a relationship.

I hope this book, and Hagrid's story, has given you some ideas, inspiration and confidence to consider various approaches to your dog's life, and to help you work with them by listening and responding to their communication.

I wish you and your animals the best of health. Enjoy each other's company, and if you have questions or would like to share your stories with me, I'd love to hear from you.

Thank you for reading,

Rosie

Further reading

TheTaleOfABigDog.com

References

Rialland, P., Bichot, S., Moreau, M. et al. Clinical validity of outcome pain measures in naturally occurring canine osteoarthritis. BMC Vet Res 8, 162 (2012). https://doi.org/10.1186/1746-6148-8-162

Kristin D. Neff, Ya-Ping Hsieh and Kullaya Dejitterat (2005) Self-compassion, Achievement Goals, and Coping with Academic Failure, Self and Identity, 4:3, 263-287, DOI: 10.1080/13576500444000317. https://self-compassion.org/wp-content/uploads/publications/SClearninggoals.pdf

Links

Rebekah Hudson:
medium.com/@theunlikelytricksters/youll-get-used-to-it-won-t-you-179933a314c2

There are some scientific studies at the end of:
wherescienceanddogsmeet.wordpress.com/2018/07/06/taking-dogs-to-the-back-of-the-veterinary-clinic-why

Vet Amber Batson makes changes for dogs:
facebook.com/story.php?story_fbid=1362950364044636&id=131337460539272

Association of British Veterinary Acupuncturists:
abva.co.uk

Lives of streeties is an observational study of Indian street dogs:
livesofstreeties.com

I agree with Linda Case about vets. The Science Dog:
thesciencedog.com/2018/02/28/be-there

Some positive changes are beginning to happen at a veterinary clinic in New York, America, who encourage carers to stay with their pets during procedures:
veg.vet

Should we reconsider the relevance of train sit?
fall2016.iaabcjournal.org/train-sit-reconsider-relevance

Robert Sapolski stress lectures are especially useful in understanding stress in humans and much of this can be applicable to understanding dogs and how their lives might be affected:
youtube.com/watch?v=NNnIGh9g6fA

Recognition of aggressive and anxious behaviours in canines by a group of Chilean veterinarians:
sciencedirect.com/science/article/abs/pii/S1558787820300435

Treats might mask animal intelligence:
sciencedaily.com/releases/2019/05/190514093420.htm

Sarah Hancox at Moorland Canine:
moorlandcanine.com

Dun Roamin animal shelter:
dun-roamin.com

Laura Dobb:
slowdogmovement.org

The gadget museum in Stratford Upon-Avon is called the MAD museum:
themadmuseum.co.uk

For more information, please visit the book's website. It includes supplemental information and links to all the further reading presented in this chapter:
thetaleofabigdog.com

Books

Understanding the silent communication of dogs (2nd edition, 2017)
by Rosie Lowry in association with Marilyn Aspinall.
Available on my website or from Amazon:
laidbackdogs.com
amazon.co.uk/gp/offer-listing/0956593410

On talking terms with dogs: Calming signals
by Turid Rugaas.
dogwise.com/on-talking-terms-with-dogs-calming-signals-2nd-edition

The Canine Thyroid Epidemic: Answers You Need for Your Dog by Jean Dodds.
dogwise.com/the-canine-thyroid-epidemic-answers-you-need-for-your-dog

Your Dog's Best Health: A Dozen Reasonable Things to Expect From Your Vet by Nancy Kay.
amazon.co.uk/gp/product/1466381957

Help Your Dog Heal Itself by Caroline Ingraham.
carolineingraham.com/store/books/help-your-dog-heal-itself-kindle-edition

Wild Health by Cindy Engel.
cindyengel.com/wild-health

There are also authors whose books have helped me find out more about holistic health, which has influenced me, my understanding, and my work with my dogs.

The following books and authors are at the foundations of my education and give me a clearer view into the lives of my dogs:

Sarah Myhill
Xandria Williams: *From Stress to Success*
Patrick Holford: *Hidden Food Allergies*
Patrick Holford: *Food is Better Medicine Than Drugs*
Anne-Lise Miller: *Too Young to Grow Old*
Dr Natasha Campbell-McBride: *Gut and Psychology Syndrome*

There are also numerous parenting books that have profoundly influenced my understanding of humans and I've been able to translate into my work with dogs:

Dan Hughes
Daniel I. Siegel, MD
Dr. Sue Gerhardt

Very important people and colleagues

Sheila Harper and Winny Boerman courses come highly recommended:
sheilaharper.com
Also look out for their forthcoming book:
Beyond Behaviour

Caroline Ingraham, zoopharmacognosy:
carolineingraham.com

Marc Bekoff:
marcbekoff.com

Jean Gough is a Dog Behaviour Advisor from Walsall (Midlands) who is knowledgeable about dogs, and her approach is gentle and empathetic; just what dogs need:
facebook.com/jean.gough.3

Sally Hopkins. Dog Games harnesses were employed for Hagrid and I use them for all dogs in my care because of the soft, evenly distributed support. A luxurious item chosen for the comfort they offer dogs:
dog-games-shop.co.uk

Miriam Krause – a vet who lives and works in the Shetland Islands:
miriamkrause.co.uk

Winkie Spiers:
winkiespiers.com

Rosee Riggs:
Austrian website: good-dog-practice.com
German website: good-dog-practice.eu

Susanne Lehr – also in Austria:
hunde-forum.at

Lisa Tenzin-Dolma – author and founder of International school for canine psychology:
theiscp.com

Andrew Hale – certified animal behaviourist:
sensitivedogs.com

Caroline Lewis – qualified dog behaviourist specialising in rescue and deaf dogs:
help-at-handdogbehaviour.com/

Martha Knowles Facebook – Silent Conversations.
A fantastic source of information for anyone wanting to learn more about the silent communication of dogs. Martha explains so well how each communication signal is used in a variety of situations:
facebook.com/silentcanineconversations
silentconversations.com/dog-body-language

Dawn Allen at Four Positive Paws:
fourpositivepaws.co.uk

Pat White:
parowhite.co.uk/sensorygarden.htm

Phil Whiteley:
leadondogbehaviour.co.uk

Pennie Clayton:
horseandhoundschool.co.uk

Julia Robertson – Galen Therapy:
galenmyotherapy.co.uk

Ann and Lyn Lowe – Design, branding and writing:
whispercreative.co.uk

Stef Dawson – Graphic/web design, content marketing and writing:
craftingwords.com

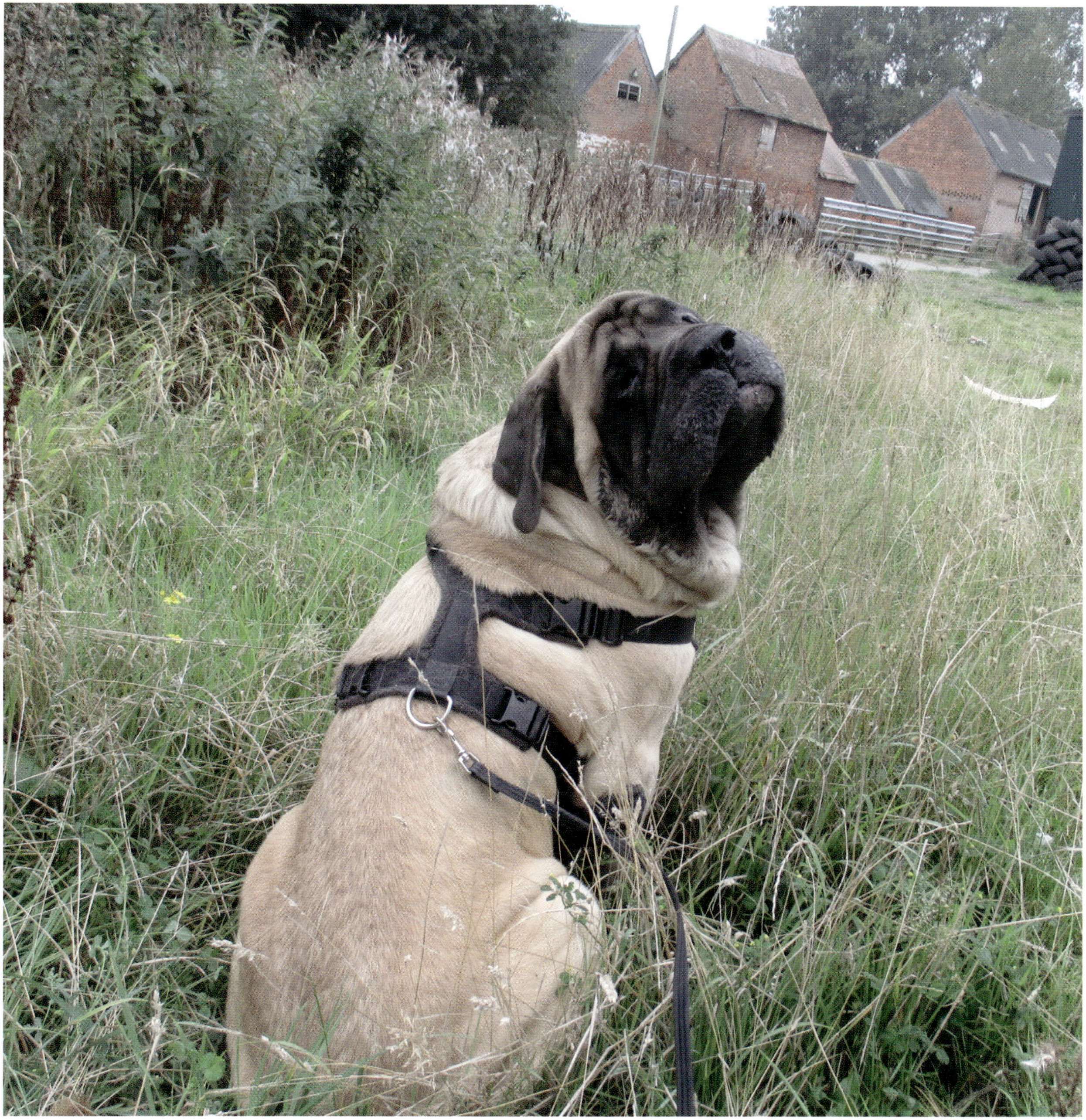

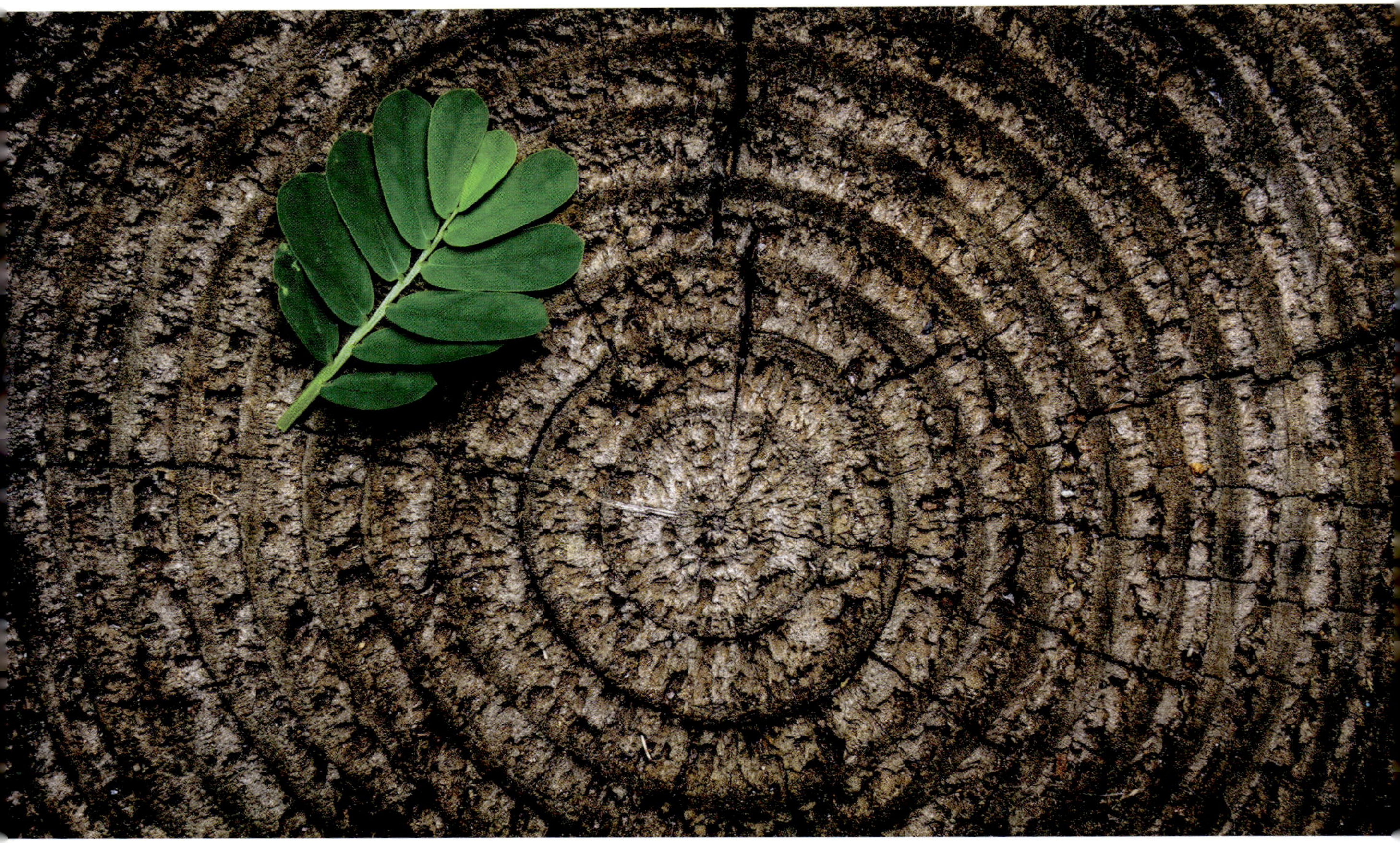

We have decided to plant a tree to celebrate Hagrid's life and to keep him alive (in a form) by scattering his ashes in the ground when planting it. We'd like your help in choosing a suitable type of tree for this, so suggestions are most welcome.

Let's see where this journey takes us and, once the tree type has been decided, chart its growth. Visit the website for more:

thetaleofabigdog.com